This concise book is an easy to read, deeply scientifically researched exploration of COVID-19. Dispels many myths and provides solid evidence for many facts. A strongly recommended read for those who want to learn more from public health scientists about the pandemic.

Jeffrey Klausner, MD, MPH, Professor of Medicine and Public Health, David Geffen School of Medicine and Fielding School of Public Health, University of California, Los Angeles

---

Facing COVID Without Panic is a short but richly educational book that is an absolute must-read for any of us – as who has not been confronting this challenging and confusing pandemic? I learned a huge amount from the "12 myths and 12 facts" that Halperin presents, and I'm sure other readers also will. Clearly explained and full of fascinating scientific data and thought-provoking tidbits. You won't be able to put it down, and your entire outlook on Covid-19 will be transformed.

Richard Wamai, PhD, Associate Professor in Public Health, Northeastern University

---

This information-packed book is a gem. It provides a clear guide to answering the questions many of us have right now about the pandemic. Should my kids go back to school? Can we visit my elderly parents? If so, how far apart do we need to be? How important is it to clean packages and other surfaces? Is it safe to go on a plane? The book does a great job at distinguishing between important measures and those that are a distraction and a waste of time.

Mark Tilton, PhD, Associate Professor of Political Science, Purdue University

---

Speaking as an editor (and a reader), I can assure you that Daniel Halperin's work is easy to read, provocative, and actionable; it brings clarity to many of the areas we have all been struggling to understand about Covid-19. At the same time, speaking both as a husband and father as well as a global public health epidemiologist, I can say confidently that ... have all faced and offers robust, evidence-grounded re ... ain and confusion, this document could not be mor ... ace)

Stephen Hodgi ...
Associate Professor of Glob ...
Editor-in-Chief, *Global* ... *Science and Practice*

Facing COVID without Panic:
12 Common Myths and 12 Lesser Known Facts about the Pandemic

Clearly Explained by an Epidemiologist

DANIEL T. HALPERIN, PhD

Gillings School of Global Public Health
University of North Carolina, Chapel Hill

To all those who grieve and have suffered from this pandemic.
And to five incredible women: my lovely daughters Leila and Ariel,
my dear mother Tam, my brave sister Dina, and my beloved Coloma.

TABLE OF CONTENTS

SUMMARY

This concise book explains in understandable terms how scientists, as they struggle to comprehend Covid-19, have begun to identify the main ways the coronavirus is spread and the primary factors associated with severe illness and death. This emerging evidence can help us determine the best ways to reduce risk as well as anxiety and fear.

By examining 12 common myths and 12 lesser known facts about Covid-19 (which are regularly updated by the author), he explores:

- How this *respiratory* coronavirus is mainly spread through close and prolonged contact, and why fleeting encounters are extremely unlikely to cause infection

- How most infections occur within *clusters* of people in indoor situations with poor air circulation: households, workplaces, nursing homes, prisons, mass transit…And what can be done about it.

- The very low risk of infection while being outdoors and from surfaces

- Why a child is more likely to die from walking to school than from Covid-19, and the surprisingly low risk of children infecting others

- Why "facial distancing" is more helpful than "social distancing"

- The value and limitations of other prevention measures including masks, gloves, thermometer guns, hand sanitizers, vaccines, 14-day quarantine periods, and "herd immunity" approaches

- Why having asthma does not increase the risk of severe illness or death from Covid-19 (and may even lower risk)

- Is it safe to work out again at the gym?

- What about "airborne" transmission: do we need to do anything differently?

- The not necessarily very high risk of old age, absent serious health conditions

- Is it safe to travel by airplane?

- The need to focus on levels of Covid-19 *deaths* (and severe illness) vs *cases*, even when surges inevitably occur

- The confusion surrounding "asymptomatic" and "pre-symptomatic" carriers

- The impact of shelter-in-place measures and other responses to the coronavirus, and

- What can be learned from past pandemics

PREFACE

I first met Dr. Daniel Halperin in 2004, while working in Zambia as a Health Advisor for the U.S. Agency for International Development (USAID). At the time, Daniel was USAID's global Primary HIV Prevention Advisor. He had come to southern Africa to provide technical assistance for supporting innovative efforts he had been developing in the region, which was and remains the world's hardest-hit by AIDS. I vividly recall attending various governmental and NGO meetings during his time in Zambia, embarrassed for him by some of the skeptical reactions, particularly from other North American and European experts in the country, to some of Daniel's then revolutionary-sounding notions about prevention. How could offering African men safe voluntary circumcision services make a dent in the raging HIV epidemic there? How would a keener understanding of complex networks of sexual culture possibly improve prevention efforts?

A little later, there was an opportunity to bring Halperin to Nepal to offer HIV prevention guidance. From my perspective, I certainly viewed Daniel as an iconoclast, but I saw real value in shaking things up. I lobbied hard but was unsuccessful. Others in the bureaucracy were more concerned with the political risks of bringing in someone with unconventional insights and an impulse to call out the Emperor wearing no clothes.

During the next few years, after clinical trials in Kenya, Uganda, and South Africa confirmed that male circumcision significantly reduced HIV transmission, and various regional consultations and conferences (largely organized by Halperin) concluded that more directly addressing sexual behavior was vital to combating AIDS, his previously controversial ideas were increasingly accepted by the UN, CDC, and other international organizations. Yet there was no basking in success for Daniel, and he continued to be a lightning rod for various sides of the political spectrum. For having believed in the value of the "Abstinence" and "Be faithful" elements of the widely-known "ABC" notion (though in Africa he mainly focused on the "B" or partner-reduction part), he often was attacked by some activists and others for being "anti-sex."

In the same year he first visited Zambia, a groundbreaking HIV prevention statement led by Halperin and published in the esteemed medical journal *The Lancet*, signed by 149 prominent scientists and global opinion leaders including Archbishop Desmond Tutu and the Ugandan President, nearly led to his dismissal by the Bush Administration because this "Common Ground" consensus document also included the "C" (for condoms) part of prevention.[1]

Although justifiably proud of these and other significant contributions while at USAID, Daniel could no longer stomach the unrelenting political mine fields; in 2007 he accepted an offer to teach and conduct research at the Harvard School of Public Health. Later, he held positions at the University of North Carolina School of Global Health (where he is currently Adjunct Full Professor), and the Ponce School of Medicine in Puerto Rico. Over this period, tiring of the politicization of the HIV/AIDS response, he shifted his focus to other pandemics facing the world, notably obesity. In early 2020, when Covid-19 struck with a vengeance – given Daniel's insatiable intellectual appetite to come to grips with what's really happening with new and complex global health challenges as well as his life-long desire to contribute to improving widespread well-being – he became caught up in the battle against this newest pandemic.

A couple of months back, as I was grappling with questions about Covid-19, I reached out to Daniel to ask how he understood the problem and learned that he'd been struggling to crystalize his own thinking in the form of a critical commentary and review of the available (yet rather incomplete) evidence. This led to him submitting a paper to the journal *Global Health: Science and Practice*,[2] of which I am Editor-in-Chief, and having the article move through our peer-review process. His paper was subsequently published in our journal.[3]

After advance publication of the article in late May of 2020, several colleagues urged him to consider making the information available to the broader public. While I do not know how this concise, valuable book will be received, I am a bit anxious that, similar to his experience many years ago – as he fought the good fight on HIV around the world – Dr. Halperin may again experience some misinformation and mischaracterization of his views. The situation indeed reminds me of the resistance he faced some 15-20 years ago, related to the inconvenient truths suggested by his insights into major drivers and potential solutions for the HIV/AIDS epidemic. When in late June he sent me an earlier version of this Covid-19 book, I saw he had made what may seem to be counter-intuitive predictions that, for example, deaths in the southern US region would probably increase somewhat during the following month, but that a surge in mortality commensurate with the soaring number of cases was unlikely to happen. In any case, there are many other lesser-known but helpful facts – and (perhaps appealing) myths – that he explores in this book, supported by the best currently available evidence. Those who decline to read it do so at their loss.

Speaking as an editor (and a reader), I can assure you that Dr. Halperin's work is easy to read, provocative, and actionable; it brings clarity to many of the areas we have all been struggling to understand about Covid-19. At the same time, speaking both as a husband and father as well as a global public health epidemiologist, I can say confidently that he addresses fears we have all faced and offers robust, evidence-grounded reassurance. After five months of pandemic pain, terror, chaos, and confusion, this document could not be more important or illuminating. I invite readers to peruse, digest, and process the information, analysis, and exceedingly useful, scientifically grounded insights he has to offer...while maintaining an open mind.

Stephen Hodgins, MD, MSc (Epidemiology & Biostatistics), DrPH, Associate Professor of Global Health, School of Public Health, University of Alberta, Canada July 9, 2020

INTRODUCTION

In early June of 2020, while finalizing a scientific article on Covid-19 for a global health journal,[3] some colleagues recommended I prepare a more accessible version for a wider audience. Particularly because many people seem anxious about how to protect themselves from the coronavirus and what measures may actually be a waste of time, I eventually agreed with my friends' suggestion. This short book is the result.

My background in public health research and programs for over four decades – half that time focused on the most recent major pandemic, HIV/AIDS[1,4,5] – to some extent prepared me for this novel pathogen. Yet I too was caught off guard by the indeed novel ways the coronavirus managed to take off around the world. I also worried about my 91-year-old mother in a senior citizens' residence in San Francisco and my sister in a nursing home there (who was hospitalized with Covid-19 in September 2020), as well as my 88-year-old Spanish mother-in-law in Madrid, one of the world's hardest-hit cities. And as this pandemic, and the response to it, began encroaching on all our lives, I had déjà vu back to those earlier years of AIDS, with the devastating number of deaths as well as the pervasive atmosphere of confusion, fear, and often panic.

In June of 1981, when the first cases were reported of what would become known as AIDS, I was living in the San Francisco Bay area. As the waves of death mounted, I eventually volunteered at a hospice in Oakland and later conducted HIV epidemiological and anthropological research at the University of California. In those early days, some political leaders were tragically slow to respond, and many, on all sides, engaged in ideological warfare, often ignoring the scientific evidence.[1,4,6] As explored in *Tinderbox*, the book I co-authored with *Washington Post* journalist Craig Timberg, even some health authorities made decisions, frequently under pressure to act quickly, that ultimately led to costly outcomes.[4,5,7] Policies would often become entrenched and difficult to walk back, even in light of new evidence. There was a tendency to defend previous decisions, and earlier openness to more innovative approaches could have saved many lives.[4-6] Well-meaning but overly simplistic messages such as "Always use a condom with anyone, or die!" inadvertently created other complications.[4,7,8] And in subsequent years, as funding began pouring in, a kind of "AIDS exceptionalism" took hold, with attention and resources for other important health problems often crowded out by the response to HIV/AIDS.[4,7,9]

During the first years of AIDS, much remained unknown about the causes and main routes of infection.[4,6,7,8] Many people understandably confused the lethality of the HIV virus (almost 100% fatal, until treatment was eventually developed) with the likelihood of infection, which is very low in most circumstances. Rumors proliferated that anything from mosquitoes to contaminated condoms to shared toothbrushes were spreading the virus. After Magic Johnson tested positive in 1991, counseling centers were overrun by the "worried well."[4,7] At a Richmond, California center where I counseled at the time, when college students and others became petrified from having engaged in deep kissing or "unprotected" intimate touching, they flooded in to get tested, diverting attention from those truly at risk of infection.

> In past health crises, authorities have often defended previous policy decisions, even in light of new evidence.

Upon immersing myself in HIV research, and later while developing prevention programs for the federal government, it often felt like I was swimming upstream against the conventional wisdom. There were seemingly endless mine fields of political ramifications and push-back along the path toward what I was convinced were more evidence-based approaches.[4,5] But eventually I realized that, as public health scientists, we have a duty not to let the present political currents outweigh evidence that can help improve people's health and well-being.[4,10] (Regarding one of the issues that many years ago caused me much grief, the role of male circumcision for HIV prevention,[4,5] while most experts were skeptical at best – and occasionally indulged in outright ridicule – one who early on recognized the scientific evidence was Anthony Fauci.[11])

With the Covid-19 pandemic, there is still much that remains unclear, with seemingly conflicting information emerging almost daily. Many of us are confused and anxious. One mindboggling indication of the level of worry is that as of May 24, 2020, the Johns Hopkins Coronavirus website was receiving some four *billion* hits a day.[12] Fear is certainly understandable, especially when spikes or occasionally large waves of new cases invariably erupt in one location or another, and fear can help motivate behavior change.[3,4,13] But irrational fear or panic often leads to impulsive decision-making and creates other problems,[14-16] for example the alarming increase in people dying this year from heart attacks and other non-Covid-19 causes due to fear of entering the hospital.[3,17-23]

Moreover, it seems we have failed to learn other important lessons from the last major pandemic, including the danger of turning a health crisis into a platform for polarized ideological point-scoring. Some politicians, media outlets, and even health experts have sought to force us into a false dichotomy, of having to choose between recklessly reopening the economy versus rigidly continuing strict lockdowns.[3,10,24,25] Reminiscent of past "condom wars," masks – a helpful complementary prevention tool when used appropriately – have become caught up in a bitter ideological battle, and judgmental attitudes such as "beach shaming" have re-emerged.[26-28] But like any pathogen, this virus does not care about politics (or national borders[29]); its only goal is how best to exploit whatever vulnerabilities we humans offer it.

> Irrational fear and panic often lead to impulsive decision-making and other negative repercussions.

Mercifully, a key difference between the new coronavirus and HIV is that, although both are RNA viruses, in the absence of treatment the coronavirus does not kill nearly everyone it infects. With Covid-19, if mainly younger persons become infected, sharp increases in new infections can occur without a correspondingly huge jump in subsequent deaths, as appears to have happened in June and July 2020 in the southern regions of the U.S. While much can be learned from responses to previous pandemics, each is, of course, different. A useful HIV strategy, like prioritizing the prevention of any new **infections**, may not be optimal for combating Covid-19, where the main focus should be on preventing severe (including longer-term) illness and **deaths** among the most vulnerable populations, such as nursing home residents.[30-32]

Recalling how well-meaning efforts to combat AIDS have occasionally led to exceptionalism and other inadvertently negative consequences,[9] the shelter-at-home and lockdown policies that saved lives by helping slow this pandemic have also led to massive repercussions, including record unemployment[24,33,34] and economic suffering[35,36] as well as dangerous increases in domestic violence,[37-39] child abuse,[40-42,146] anxiety and depression,[40,43-45] drug overdoses,[46] obesity,[47,48] and divorces.[49] We are still learning how to take useful precautions for avoiding risk, without falling into panic or despair or counterproductive efforts that may create more harm than good.

It is worth repeating that this truly is a *novel* virus. Hence there are many aspects, including some of the "myths" and "facts" explored below, about which scientists still know relatively little or are uncertain. Furthermore, this is not an everything-about-coronaviruses book. And as researchers continue discovering and clarifying more evidence on a daily basis, I plan to update this living document at regular intervals and, when possible, to address questions, concerns or issues posed by readers.

12 COMMON MYTHS

■ **MYTH 1:** Covid-19 is really no worse than the annual flu.

Although some politicians and even a few researchers initially thought this might be the case, Covid-19 appears to be at least five times more lethal than the seasonal flu. Based on large antibody surveys that identify people who previously have been infected with the coronavirus, the actual fatality rate (which for various reasons is very difficult to estimate[50-52]) seems to be roughly in the range of 0.2-1%, meaning that somewhere between 1 in 500 to about 1 in 100 persons who become infected will die.[50,53] In June 2020 the CDC estimated a fatality rate of 0.26%, yet the following month a World Health Organization (WHO) panel concurred on an estimate of 0.64%.[51,52]

Of course, the chances of dying are much greater in older and sicker persons, and far lower in younger and healthier ones. University of Cambridge statistician Sir David Spiegelhalter has observed that in women in the U.K. aged 30-34, "around 1 in 70,000 died from Covid-19 over the 9 peak weeks of the epidemic. Since over 80% of these had preexisting medical conditions, we estimate that healthy women in this age-group had less than a 1 in 350,000 risk of dying from Covid, around 1/4 of the normal risk of an accidental death over this period."[54] Meanwhile, the actual fatality rate of influenza, which also mainly affects older and other vulnerable people, appears to be less than 0.1%, although the annual flu kills more infants and young children than Covid-19.[55]

> Covid-19 is at least 5 times more lethal than the seasonal flu (but more children die from the flu).

■ **MYTH 2:** This pandemic is nearly as bad as the Spanish Flu a century ago.

Thankfully, this also is not true. That horrific pandemic slaughtered around 50 million people, when the world's population was less than a fourth of what it is today. The fatality rate of the "Spanish Flu" was probably five to ten times greater than that of Covid-19, and it killed many healthy young adults and children; the average age of death is estimated to have been 28.[56,57] In contrast, Covid-19 overwhelmingly affects the elderly, especially those with serious health conditions. The average (median) age of Covid-19-related deaths has been in the low to mid-80s in European countries and about 80 in the U.S.[58]

> The vast majority of deaths occur in persons with an underlying chronic condition like diabetes or obesity.

Between 96% (in the U.S.) and 99% (in Italy) of deaths, at any age, have occurred in persons with one or more of certain preexisting chronic diseases such as diabetes and heart or kidney disease,[59-61] with those (especially men) who are obese[62-64] or who smoke[65,66] at twice or greater risk.

■ **MYTH 3:** It is easy to become infected through casual contact.

With Covid-19 there has been a tendency, as happened with HIV, to confuse the new virus's potential *lethality* with its *contagiousness*. This is understandable, especially when the pandemic seemingly is spreading out of control. And infection from the coronavirus certainly is quite possible, normally much more so than with HIV. As with other *respiratory* pathogens, this is particularly the case if your *face* maintains relatively *close* and *prolonged* exposure (probably for at least about 15 minutes) to the *face* of an infected person.[3,67-69] Transmission is especially likely if a contagious individual coughs, sneezes, shouts, or sings forcefully in your direction. However, if you are in sufficiently close (less than about 3 feet) and prolonged contact, particularly indoors, the infectious droplets emitted during normal speaking and breathing can be enough to cause infection.

Along with other infectious diseases, scientists believe there is a "dose response" for Covid-19, meaning the combination of *intensity* and *duration* of exposure predicts the likelihood of contagion (and probably eventual clinical outcomes).[67,68,70,71] This involves a threshold – or a *minimum amount of viral particles* – required to cause infection. The concept of dose response helps explain, for example, the extremely low risk from fleeting encounters, such as momentarily walking past someone, since this is very unlikely to entail a sufficiently intense or prolonged exposure to result in infection. Dose response probably also helps explain the large number of medical workers who have been severely affected by Covid-19, since they tend to be in close and relatively extended contact with symptomatic and often very sick individuals.[68,70]

> **The risk from simply walking past someone or briefly exchanging hugs is extremely low, as such events are very unlikely to involve a sufficient level of viral exposure.**

As with other serious health concerns, practicing evidence-based precautions is crucial. Yet it is also vital for one's mental health and quality of life not to suffer from becoming anxious or fearful, disproportionately to the actual risk.[3,14-16,27,67,71] For example, scientifically speaking there is little reason to refrain from giving hugs, as long as you avoid prolonged face-to-face proximity.

■ MYTH 4: Contaminated surfaces are an important means of infection and require meticulous precautions.

Laboratory experiments have found that the coronavirus can survive for up to several days on hard surfaces such as elevator buttons, doorknobs, and countertops. Yet based on the available evidence for viral transmission, as the CDC has concluded (and similarly to other respiratory infections) the *actual risk appears to be very low.*[72-74] Considering the large number of customers served by industries such as transportation, rigorous sterilization procedures have been adopted by airlines, taxi services, and hotels (although the standard Covid-19-related practice of only renting out rooms that have been left vacant for several days is not scientifically warranted). Yet in ordinary circumstances, including at home, the actual likelihood of infection does not warrant the obsessive attention to disinfection often being performed.

Emanuel Goldman, a Professor of Microbiology, Biochemistry and Molecular Genetics at New Jersey Medical School, summarized the available data in a July 2020 paper in the medical journal *The Lancet*.[72] As Dr. Goldman explains: "The problem with those experiments was that the amount of virus they started with was much, much orders of magnitude larger than what you're going to find in the real world."[73] He notes that some studies measured the virus's lifespan by placing as much as "a hundred thousand to 10 million virus particles on a small surface area," vastly greater than the amount of virus present in a human sneeze. Dr. Goldman is concerned that "The supermarkets won't take returns of anything that you buy now because of this…And it's in ways little and large that it's directed behaviour that's not justified by the data."[73]

The renowned University of Minnesota coronavirus expert Michael Osterholm corroborates: "The public right now is so confused about what is safe and what's not safe. And one of the challenges has been this idea that surfaces play a major role in transmission. We've looked very carefully at the data, dating back for decades and research about these kinds of respiratory transmitted infections. And clearly, the surfaces play a very, very little role at all in transmission of this. I think we've gone way overboard relative to the disinfection and so forth, and we've made people feel very nervous about just opening a package…I mean, this is really all about breathing someone else's air where the virus is present. It's much, much, much less about environmental contamination."[71]

> Coronavirus expert Osterholm: "I think we've gone way overboard, we've made people feel very nervous about just opening a package…I mean, this is about air."

Moreover, because the coronavirus can potentially cause death, not surprisingly many assume bleach or other strong cleaning products are necessary to kill it. As a result, *toxic reactions and hospitalizations from misuse of such products have soared.*[16,75] In fact, normal use of soap and water or household detergent, as recommended by the CDC, are perfectly adequate to eliminate the coronavirus.[74,76] Wearing gloves may actually increase risk, including because the virus tends to remain on latex.[77,78] Good hand washing practices are much more important.[76] The FDA has strongly warned against using certain hand sanitizers containing the lethal ingredient methanol.[79] Indeed, the widespread use of these alcohol-based sanitizing products is unnecessary in many instances, where soap and water are readily available, and in some people they cause skin irritation and other issues.[76] Many (also overly used) antibacterial wipes are only effective, as the name implies, with bacteria and not with viruses.[80,81]

Although thermometer guns may be useful in areas with high Covid-19 prevalence, their increasingly routine utilization in low-prevalence settings, where a high temperature much more likely results from any number of other reasons, is certainly questionable.[82] One laboratory study created a stir by suggesting that fecal particles containing the coronavirus can enter the surrounding air, due to the flushing action, and potentially cause infection.[83,84] However, as experts such as Osterholm have cautioned, we should avoid giving too much credence to preliminary and often non-peer-reviewed studies, some of which are finding the spotlight during a time of intensified public concern.[71] (However, *if* empirical research were to actually confirm that hypothetical possibility, perhaps governments should consider mandating lids be added to public toilets where needed.)

Many scientists and the public are increasingly concerned about the potential for aerosol-based infection, i.e., the coronavirus's ability to linger in the air or possibly move across relatively large distances, especially in indoor settings with poor ventilation. Although some data suggest this could be a factor in transmission to health workers, particularly while engaged in respiratory procedures such as intubation and administrating medication by nebulizer, as the WHO reports there is so far insufficient evidence to confirm this transmission mode is prevalent in community settings.[85] Similarly to the low risk of surface transmission, it may be that the amount of viral particles released into the air is normally inadequate to cause infection. Yet this area of concern urgently requires further study and analysis to inform practical conclusions and potential policy decisions.

A July 2020 review of the evidence for aerosol transmission made a parallel to the earlier heightened fears regarding the risk from surface contamination, concluding that, "As the science comes in, recommendations can be fine-tuned based on what we learn. In the meantime, there is no reason to be any more alarmed or even, in most cases, to change what we're doing to protect ourselves and others."[86] However, the real possibility that aerosol transmission is a significant risk factor reinforces the ongoing importance of taking additional precautions in indoor settings with poor circulation and ventilation of air.[3,67,71] (Fortunately, the risk of traveling by airplane appears to be much lower than was assumed, thanks to the effectiveness of the air circulation and filtration systems used on commercial flights.[87])

> The potential risk of aerosol transmission reinforces the importance of taking precautions in indoor settings with poor air circulation and ventilation.

■ MYTH 5: Asymptomatic persons are a major driver of the pandemic.

Despite much speculation and some modeling exercises, empirical research to date suggest that persons who are "asymptomatic," meaning those who will never develop symptoms, are probably rarely contagious.[88-90] When a WHO scientist referred to these data on June 8, 2020, the global agency was hit by an avalanche of criticism not only because more research is needed, but because the confusion created by the remark might inadvertently have called into question the value of wearing masks.[91] Much of the attack on the WHO referenced a widely cited review article that curiously asserted (based on two or three Italian persons who "may" have been infected by asymptomatic individuals) that such carriers are important pandemic spreaders.[92] Indicative of the ongoing confusion related to this disease's complexity, the authors' more evidence-based conclusion that up to 40-45% of all those *infected* by the coronavirus are asymptomatic was misunderstood by some commentators as meaning that nearly half of all *infections* are due to asymptomatic transmission.

Another important reason for the confusion surrounding the WHO controversy involves the distinction between asymptomatic carriers and those who are "pre-symptomatic," meaning they have not yet but will develop symptoms within the next several days.[88-90] While it is pretty clear that infection does occur from pre-symptomatic individuals, such pre-symptomatic yet contagious persons comprise relatively few carriers at any given moment, considering the short time duration (usually less than 48 hours) in this phase. Furthermore, many appear to have low "viral loads," which would help explain why: 1) they don't yet have symptoms; 2) many may receive a negative result from the standard PCR coronavirus test,[93] and 3) research to date suggests they are likely to be less contagious than actively symptomatic persons.[88-90]

In an analysis of 243 Covid-19 cases in Singapore, 6% appeared to originate from pre-symptomatic carriers.[94] Some other examples of pre-symptomatic transmission have also been reported.[89,92,95] Although high viral loads have been detected in some pre-symptomatic carriers, the implications for the pandemic's spread are unclear.[70,96] With HIV, for example, viral load is strongly associated with infectivity, but the fact that pre-symptomatic coronavirus carriers are not actively coughing or sneezing may largely explain their lower contagiousness, compared to infected persons who have such symptoms. In reality, viral load often may not be particularly important for transmission – and therefore in spreading the pandemic –

among persons who are not actively symptomatic. That said, if they maintain close and prolonged proximity, or are shouting, singing or otherwise forcefully expelling infectious droplets over a greater distance, pre-symptomatic individuals (especially those with higher viral loads) can certainly transmit the coronavirus. More research is needed, but the existing evidence does at least suggest there is considerably higher likelihood of transmission from those late in the pre-symptomatic phase than from carriers who will never develop symptoms.[89,90] Nonetheless, the

WHO's assessment that asymptomatic and pre-symptomatic persons are unlikely to be very important drivers of Covid-19's spread[88] so far appears to be correct, although the potential role of pre-symptomatic transmission should not be ignored.

> Viral load may not be very important for transmission, and therefore in spreading the pandemic, among persons who aren't symptomatic.

■ MYTH 6: Wearing masks is always necessary.

If worn by *infected* persons, cloth-type masks provide you *some* protection in circumstances of *close* and relatively *prolonged* proximity, especially in enclosed indoor spaces. Similar to other public health measures, this however can be taken to an extreme. As former CDC Director Thomas Frieden has observed, scientifically there is no reason to wear a mask if you are not near anyone else,[97] such as while strolling or driving alone.[71] In fact, strict enforcement of mask-wearing, including in situations where it is not justifiable for prevention purposes, may exacerbate other health problems.[98,99] Wearing them for protracted periods, as many workers are now required to do even if not in close contact with other persons, can be very uncomfortable, especially in hot weather.

Extended mask-wearing has caused some elderly and other persons with breathing difficulties to faint or even require hospitalization, for example while waiting in the sun to enter stores that severely restrict the numbers of customers

> Scientifically, there is no reason to wear a mask if you are not near anyone else, such as while driving or strolling alone.

allowed inside.[3,98,99] Furthermore, experts caution about the common problem of incorrect placement, as well as the false sense of security potentially created by wearing masks, which are only partially protective, that may lead to neglect of other important precautions such as hygiene and distancing.[100] *It is better to be located a safe distance away from infected persons who are not using masks than to be near them, even if wearing masks.*

Perhaps reminiscent of some hurriedly-adopted and ultimately misguided past AIDS policies, Michael Osterholm (who supports appropriate mask-wearing) criticizes the lack of solid data for the effectiveness of cloth masks to support the CDC's abrupt May 2020 policy reversal: "Never before in my 45-year career have I seen such a far-reaching public recommendation issued by any governmental agency…This is an extremely worrisome precedent of implementing policies not based on science-based data or why they were issued without such data."[101]

However, while awaiting more conclusive evidence, in situations where sufficient distance cannot be maintained from other people's faces, including visits to doctors or barbers or while using mass transit and airplanes, some studies have shown cloth-type masks to reduce the likelihood of transmitting the coronavirus.[102] They may also partially protect against becoming infected (and importantly, may reduce the risk of severe outcomes if infected), an issue requiring more rigorous evaluation.[103] N-95 surgical masks are much more effective, but of course need to be prioritized for health care professionals and others at high risk, and those which include a release valve only reduce the wearer's risk of infection but do not protect others if the user is infected.[101] Although as discussed asymptomatic and pre-symptomatic carriers may only be responsible for a relatively minor proportion of total infections, pending further research and in populations where the coronavirus is circulating widely, a universal norm of wearing cloth masks in crowded (especially indoors) settings is a useful complementary public health measure.[71,97]

■ MYTH 7: "Social distancing" of at least six feet is always necessary.

As mentioned previously and as with other respiratory infections, close and prolonged proximity with someone who may be infected, especially indoors, should be avoided whenever possible. In early 2020 the WHO and European and Asian health authorities recommended physical distancing based on identification of infectious droplets almost a meter (about three feet) away from coughing and sneezing individuals.[104] Meanwhile, in the U.S. one meter was initially translated into five feet and subsequently became "over six feet." Such an abundance-of-caution expansion of international standards may make sense in certain situations, and arguably a hard-and-fast rule to "always stay over 6 feet away from anyone" is simpler to mandate.

However, scientifically it is unclear whether this is necessary, especially for *outdoor* (see Fact #3) commercial and recreational activities including construction, landscaping, playgrounds, and terrace dining. It is clearly more practical to maintain a distance of about three feet instead of over six feet in situations such as grocery shopping, where interactions are typically very brief, or while strolling outdoors with a companion.[3] As a June 2020 review recommended, "A graded approach to physical distancing that reflects the individual setting, the indoor space and air condition, and other protective factors may be the best approach to reduce risk."[105]

Many commentators have criticized the term "social distancing," since maintaining social connections is more important than ever,[71,106-108] particularly as mental health problems related to isolation have soared.[8,14-16,40,45,46] In fact, the concept of "physical" distancing is also not directly related to how the coronavirus is mainly spread: via *respiratory* droplets.[3,67,68,71] What is actually most relevant is the distance between people's **faces**, not the distance between their **bodies**. For example, if persons in a restaurant or office are seated back-to-back, a safe distance can be considerably closer than if they are positioned face-to-face. (However, in indoor settings with poor ventilation, especially given the potential importance of aerosol transmission, maintaining a greater distance would be prudent.) And if someone facing in your direction may be actively symptomatic, keeping over six feet of distance is certainly a good idea. Meanwhile, if a jogger or bicyclist zooms past you, transmission is almost impossible, since the droplets scatter and evaporate quickly and because, as discusssed earlier, such fleeting interactions are very unlikely to lead to infection. In any case, a concept such as "facial distancing" could be more useful than "social" or "physical" distancing.

> What counts is the distance between people's **faces**, not their **bodies**. If people are seated back-to-back, a safe distance is considerably closer than if they're face-to-face.

■ MYTH 8: Children are at considerable risk of getting very ill or dying from Covid-19, and are super-spreaders who can easily infect other kids and adults.

Despite the widespread attention given to a disturbing "Kawasaki"-like acute inflammatory syndrome associated with Covid-19, severe illness and death from this SARS-2 coronavirus, as with the first SARS epidemic in 2002-03,[109,110] have been extremely uncommon in young persons.[3,111-113] Among the few hundred children worldwide so far known to have contracted this inflammatory syndrome, nearly all have recovered within weeks, as happens with the usual Kawasaki disease, especially if detected and treated early.[114] Of the over 450,000 deaths reported globally as of late June 2020, some two dozen were among persons under the age of 18, about half of them in the U.S.[111,113,115] By comparison, for *each* known Covid-19 child death in the U.S., about 20 kids died last year from the flu, nearly 100 from drownings, and about 200 in car accidents.[116] According to the aforementioned statistician Sir David Spiegelhalter, "If you're aged 5-14 and you haven't had it yet, your chance of death from Covid is 1 in 3,579,551. You are more likely to die walking to school."[117]

> For every child who's died of Covid-19, about 20 will die from the flu, 100 from drownings, and 200 in car accidents.

An emerging body of biological and epidemiological evidence indicates that, unlike other respiratory pathogens such as the common cold, but similar to the earlier SARS-1 virus, children are both less likely to become infected with and less able to transmit the new SARS coronavirus.[96,112,113,115,118-120] According to the CDC, as of May 2020 only 1.7% of all U.S. Covid-19 cases had been reported in persons aged 18 years or younger.[121] Scientists have discovered that children are less easily infected because of lower production of the ACE-2 protein, the key (nasal) entry point for both SARS coronaviruses.[110,115,122] Furthermore, it is believed that previous exposure to the common cold coronaviruses frequently acquired by children may provide some partial immunity to the new variant.[96,115,123] Intriguingly, when blood samples collected before 2019 were analyzed (i.e., before humans were first exposed to Covid-19), about half those studied already appeared to have had some protective immunity to the new SARS virus, apparently due to past exposure to other coronaviruses.[123]

Moreover, available evidence suggests that even when children do become infected, they are less contagious than adults.[96,112,113,115,118,119,120] In July 2020, South Korean researchers reported that *symptomatic* children ages 10-19 appeared to be even more contagious than adults.[124] However, doubts have been raised about this finding, including the possibility that many children may have been infected by adults, rather than the other way around.[125] Crucially, and also absent from most of the widespread discussion of this study, only 2% of all (symptomatic) persons identified were in that age range, and less than 1% of 54,000 contacts traced by the researchers were ages 10-19.[124] Consistent with this data, a June 2020 *Nature* study found that 79% of infected persons ages 10-19 were asymptomatic.[126]

Another widely cited study concluded that viral load levels in infected children are comparable to those in adults, although this preliminary finding has been called into question by Spiegelhalter and others.[96,127,128] Even among youth with high viral levels in their nasal tracks, *if lacking symptoms such as coughing or sneezing they will expel far fewer infectious droplets.*[70,96] Indeed, contact tracing studies conducted in China, Iceland, the U.K., the Netherlands, and some other countries could not identify a single instance of child-to-adult transmission out of many thousands of cases analyzed.[96,112,115,119,120,129] A review of household infection studies from several Asian countries concluded that less than 10% of family clusters involved a child bringing the coronavirus into the home.[130]

> In a widely cited Korean study, **symptomatic persons ages 10-19 seemed more contagious, but only 2% of infected individuals were in that age group.**

Of course, when reopening schools careful precautions must be taken for protecting students, teachers, and other school employees.[112,131,132] And parents and others should be prepared for the occasional flareups of cases that will inevitably occur, knowing these will not necessarily – and in fact are unlikely to – lead to major epidemic eruptions. Those countries that never closed schools or reopened them by mid-May 2020, including Denmark,[133] Norway, New Zealand, France, Germany, Netherlands, Taiwan, Finland, and Vietnam, have not experienced national increases in new Covid-19 cases or deaths.[134-136] An April 2020 evaluation of data from five primary schools and ten high schools in Australia found that although nine staff members and nine students had been infected, no other staff or teachers and only two additional students may have subsequently become infected, even though those 18 infected persons had been in daily contact with 735 other students and 128 staff members.[137]

A study conducted in a high-prevalence region of France, involving 540 schoolchildren ages 6-11 and 42 teachers, identified no instances of children infecting other children or adults.[138] German researchers who tested 1,500 high school students and 500 teachers in May/June 2000 found very few had been infected, concluding that schoolchildren could even be "acting as a brake on infection" at the population level.[139] In the U.S., a preliminary analysis of some 40,000 children who remained in YMCA child care centers, including 10,000 in New York City, identified very few secondary infections (no more than one per site).[140,141] In a separate study of 916 day care centers involving more than 20,000 children, only about 1% of staff and 0.16% of children had been infected.[140] (It is unclear whether those persons were infected at the centers or elsewhere.)

> Keeping schools closed is exacerbating socioeconomic disparities, as children from disadvantaged backgrounds fall perilously behind.

The repercussions of keeping children at home have been enormous, *particularly in lower-income communities*, including undoubtedly long-lasting academic setbacks for many millions of students.[142,143] Moreover, there have been dangerous increases in social isolation,[40,43] both hunger and obesity due to missed subsidized lunches and school-related physical exercise,[47,48,118,144,145] and child abuse.[40,41,42,146] Additionally, socioeconomic disparities are exacerbated, as some families have the technological tools, parental academic assistance, and other resources to enhance online learning, while less privileged children fall perilously behind.[130,145,147,148] All of this makes it increasingly difficult, as the American Academy of Pediatrics concluded in June 2020, to justify stopping some 55 million children in the U.S. (and hundreds of millions worldwide) from returning to their classrooms.[112]

Students with special needs such as autism, Downs syndrome, and ADHD are at particular risk, though months away from friends and the daily routine of classes has taken a toll on all children, as beleaguered parents everywhere can attest.[131,142,147,149] Disturbingly, in large surveys young people report far higher levels of both anxiety and depression than do other age groups (with older Americans curiously reporting the lowest levels).[44,45] In a national CDC survey conducted in late June, 75% of 18-to-24 years olds reported experiencing anxiety and/or depression (three times levels in 2019), with 25% saying they had thought about suicide during the previous 30 days.[45] In any case, as evidence regarding children and Covid-19 continues to emerge and

> Students with special needs like autism and ADHD are at highest risk, but months away from friends and a daily routine hurt all kids.

become more widely disseminated, parents will of course need to decide what is in the best interests of their own families, and teachers and other school employees likewise should have the right to assess risk and other factors.[112,131,142,145]

■ MYTH 9: Simply being older or having asthma or HIV puts you at much higher risk of becoming seriously ill or dying from Covid-19.

While more evidence is being collected and analyzed, raw statistics suggest that an 85-year-old person not suffering from specific underlying medical conditions such as serious heart or kidney disease, diabetes, or obesity may be at lower risk of dying from Covid-19 than a 55-year-old who has at least one (and especially several) such conditions. The fact that older persons on average are at much greater risk of dying may largely be due to the elderly being much more likely to have such preexisting chronic illnesses. In addition, there might be biological reasons why persons older than about 65 are more likely to become *infected*, including possibly greater production of the aforementioned ACE-2 protein entry point.[110,121]

Furthermore, there very likely are reasons, particularly immune system decline, why simply being elderly also increases the risk of dying from the disease. But considering that the vast majority of Covid-19 deaths, *at any age*, occur in persons with certain underlying serious medical problems,[59-61] the increased risk of old age by itself may not be nearly as dramatic as has been commonly assumed.[58] More research and analysis would better determine the independently increased risk from being elderly, in the absence of preexisting health conditions. In addition, quality of life concerns are vitally important, such as feeling comfortable briefly hugging one's grandchildren, which Swiss health authorities have encouraged since this is not inherently risky.[150]

....

Because asthma is also a respiratory condition, intuitively it would seem to increase risk for complications from Covid-19. It is therefore not surprising that many people with the ailment, including many young persons, have been frightened of becoming very ill or dying if they get infected. Such anxiety has at times led to shortages of inhalers and other critical supplies. Yet investigators examining the association between asthma and serious Covid-19 outcomes or deaths found no such link,[151] and subsequent research has confirmed this finding.[152-154] On June 25, 2020, the CDC modified its website to state that having moderate to severe asthma "might be" (rather than "is"[3,154]) a risk factor for severe Covid-19 outcomes.

In fact, scientists are perplexed because some evidence suggests having asthma might even be somewhat *protective*.[153] For example, data from New York indicate only 5% of Covid-19 deaths were among people with asthma, even though they comprise 8% of the population at large.[152] Persons with allergic asthma appear to produce less ACE-2 protein, and researchers are also investigating whether standard allergy medications such as inhaled corticosteroids may partially prevent severe Covid-19 complications.[153] There is also understandable concern about persons co-infected with both HIV and the coronavirus. An Italian study found they do not experience more severe outcomes from Covid-19 compared to HIV-negative persons.[155] However, a South African study found a relatively modest increased risk of death for persons with both HIV and Covid-19.[156]

■ MYTH 10: Increases in *cases* inevitably lead to corresponding increases in *deaths*.

Although the media, politicians, and even many experts habitually imply that rises in new *cases* are by definition a disaster – as opposed to spikes in severe illness and *deaths*, which of course *are* a tragedy – it is critical to remember that as testing expands, more cases will also inevitably be identified.[157] More importantly, a comparison of death rates between different countries rather dramatically shows how the number of reported cases does not inexorably equate with a similarly corresponding level of deaths. The number of deaths compared to reported cases, or the case-fatality rate, in such countries as South Korea (2.3% on June 22, 2020), Germany (4.5%), Norway (2.8%), Denmark (4.8%), and Japan (5.3%) has been much lower than in nations including Italy (14%), France (16%), Belgium (16%), and the U.K. (14%).[158] (Case fatality rates are nearly always far greater than *actual* fatality rates, which as previously mentioned are more precisely determined via large-scale, population-based antibody surveys.[50-52,159])

The lower mortality in places such as Germany has partly been due to use of more effective treatment methods. Yet the primary reason for the lower death rates in certain countries is that – as of mid-May 2020, by when the vast majority of Covid-19 deaths in Europe and Asia had occurred – relatively more younger persons had become infected, compared to those countries with higher mortality rates, where rela*tively many more cases had been reported among the elderly.*[160] (In addition, testing rates have been higher in countries including Germany and South Korea, where the total number of reported cases is therefore also greater, although in Japan, for example, testing has not been widespread).

One implication of this evidence is that we should not automatically assume that a higher number of cases equals correspondingly greater levels of serious illness and death. This is a rather different situation compared to other epidemics, such as HIV before treatment, when more infections did invariably translate over time into a commensurate increase in deaths. With Covid-19, *if mainly younger and healthier people are infected then proportionally far less severe illness and death will result.* An important conclusion is that we ought not to have focused so much on, for example, reprimanding college students for frolicking on beaches.[27] (As Michael Osterholm notes, beaches are, "ironically, probably some of the safest places to go to if you're not literally cheek and jowl with someone."[71]) Rather than berating people for such low-risk activities, if we had targeted prevention efforts much more towards carefully protecting long-term elderly care residents – ideally through wiser approaches than just tightly locking down these facilities indefinitely – as well as preventing infections among other high-risk groups such as meatpacking plant workers, prison inmates and guards, then many more lives could have been saved.

While blame games over the past are unhelpful, going forward it is imperative to prioritize prevention efforts strategically targeting the most vulnerable among us. This should include policy measures such as better remuneration and protection for nursing home employees. A significant part of the mortality in such institutions, especially among those that suffered an unusually large number of deaths, appears to have been from clinical "abandonment" of patients due to acute staffing shortages, exacerbated by fear of contracting the virus.[31,161] A key take-home lesson is that for every 10,000 Covid-19 cases prevented among residents of elderly care homes (such as through improving air ventilation systems), **vastly more** hospitalizations and deaths will be avoided than by preventing 10,000 new infections in college-age youth.

> For every 10,000 Covid-19 cases prevented among nursing home residents, vastly more deaths will be avoided than by preventing 10,000 infections in college-age youth.

■ MYTH 11: Getting infected is (always) a very bad thing.

Not necessarily. The large majority of people infected with this coronavirus, especially younger and healthier ones, will suffer relatively few symptoms and many will have none at all, the latter being those asymptomatic carriers who may comprise nearly half of all infected persons.[92,123] Within two weeks following initial exposure, probably most infected persons will at least to a large extent have been "naturally vaccinated." Experts including Anthony Fauci had generally believed that immunity probably extends for up to a year or more.[162] Yet in July 2020 researchers in Spain and the U.K. reported that antibodies in many people appear to diminish quickly over a relatively short period (worrisomely suggesting that potential vaccines might also only work for a short duration).[163-165] However, other emerging data, including on the importance of different functions of the immune system such as "memory" T-cells, suggest that immunity is probably longer-lasting, though clearly the issue is not yet fully resolved.[123,164,165]

Assuming that relatively long-lasting immunity is indeed created, already-infected persons may be able to return to work or school with presumably much lower risk of (re)infection, perhaps including safely being near older and other vulnerable persons. However, there have been cases, which thankfully are statistically rare despite being highlighted by the media, of young and healthy people requiring hospitalization or even dying, so we must not assume there is *no* risk from becoming infected. Furthermore, while the great majority of persons who survive will recover within a couple of weeks, quite a few will suffer an extremely unpleasant experience.[166] Even more disturbingly, an apparently considerable number of people will continue to have symptoms, often quite severe ones, for an extended period,[167-169] an emerging issue that researchers and clinicians are urgently investigating.[166,168-170] (With other respiratory illnesses including influenza, a range of long-term severe complications is also not uncommon.[171]) And of course, those infected with the coronavirus should first be quarantined to avoid infecting others.

One international standard that may eventually be worth revisiting regards the period of time required for routinely quarantining persons for various reasons, including having arrived from another country or

> Some people will continue to have symptoms, occasionally quite severe ones, for an extended period.

area. (The latter policy is increasingly being criticized by leading scientists.[29,172]) It may be that the standard 14-day wait period constitutes an overabundance of caution, considering that: 1) the average length of time before developing Covid-19 symptoms is 5-6 days,[173] 2) a May 2020 study found that 98% of symptomatic carriers developed symptoms by 11 days,[173,174] and 3) as previously discussed, studies to date suggest asymptomatic and pre-symptomatic carriers are considerably less contagious.[88-90] Perhaps a group of objective experts might end up concluding that, for example, a 10-day period is statistically/epidemiologically reasonable, if practical implications would merit changing the policy. Indeed, in September 2020 some European countries such as France began debating whether to reduce the quarantine period to as short as five days.

. . . .

Meanwhile, some countries like Sweden had contemplated adopting a controversial strategy of attempting to reach "herd immunity," i.e., essentially allowing younger and healthier people to remain at or gradually return to work and school, assuming that in the process many could become infected.[24,175-177] The concept is based on the premise that if roughly 60% of the population eventually becomes infected, and thereby naturally immunized (presuming that relatively long-lasting immunity is conferred) the virus would then have much more difficulty in finding new hosts and would ultimately recede, even in the absence of a medical vaccine (which some researchers fear might take several more years to successfully develop[178]).

Antibody testing conducted in New York City found as many as 68% of people in some lower-income neighborhoods had previously been infected, compared to under 15% in more affluent areas.[179] Even if a lesser amount, for example 30% of the population, becomes infected this probably means that considerably fewer people will be vulnerable to a future wave of infection.[180] An international group of mathematicians has even calculated that, under certain circumstances, a threshold as low as surprisingly only 20% might be sufficient to create herd immunity.[181] If this unusual hypothesis proves to have some merit, it may help explain why by mid-July 2020 the earlier epicenters of infection – New York, Detroit, Madrid, Milan, etc. – had yet to see indications of a resurgence in new cases.[181] Importantly, part of the reason for a possibly lower herd immunity threshold may be the aforementioned widespread degree of partial immunity evidently caused by previous exposure to other coronaviruses.[123,164,165,180,181]

Large-scale antibody testing, which several other countries have also begun implementing, could enhance herd-immunity approaches, although the accuracy and reliability of these tests for clinical purposes has occasionally been problematic.[50,71,159,182] In any case, interest may eventually grow in alternatives to continually trying to stamp out all new infections, which in places including China and Germany has turned into a whack-a-mole challenge.[183] Although clearly imperfect, something along the lines of a herd immunity approach might emerge as a more realistic, least-terrible, longer-term alternative, perhaps including in some lower-income regions with comparatively much younger populations.[3,184-186] In such settings, even if widespread transmission occurs it would likely result in *considerably fewer per-capita deaths than in places with many more elderly persons.*[187-189] Crucially, we must determine how best to protect those most vulnerable people, particularly the elderly with certain preexisting medical conditions – certainly no easy task. Consideration of alternatives to lockdowns including herd immunity-based approaches may intensify if a major wave occurs in late 2020 or early 2021, although as mentioned such controversial strategies could be far from ideal.

■ **MYTH 12:** In places like Sweden that did not lock down their economies and societies, there have been more deaths from Covid-19.

The media as well as some experts have highlighted the higher official death rate in Sweden compared to other Scandinavian countries, which as discussed have reported (along with some other countries including Germany, South Korea, and Japan) unusually low mortality rates relative to elsewhere in Europe and the U.S.[3,158,190,191] But as experts such as Thomas Frieden have urged, rather than relying on official tallies of Covid-19 death rates, which are often notoriously incomplete, it is usually preferable to determine numbers of "excess" deaths, through comparing current mortality to levels from previous years.[157,192-194] Cross-country comparisons of government statistics and numbers of excess deaths reveal that while official Covid-19 mortality tabulations in a handful of nations including

> Excess deaths in Sweden have been lower than in many other places, including Italy, Spain, Belgium, Holland, the U.S., Peru, Ecuador, and the U.K., all of which, unlike Sweden, imposed strict lockdowns.

Belgium and Sweden have captured nearly all excess deaths, most countries have significantly missed the mark, under-reporting by as much as 88% of excess deaths.[3,193,194] As of August 28, the number of per-capita excess deaths since early 2020 was lower in Sweden than in over a dozen other places, including Italy, Spain, Belgium, the Netherlands, the U.S., Ecuador, Peru, Chile, and the U.K., all of which, unlike Sweden, imposed strict lockdowns.[190,191,193,194]

However, while daily Covid-19 deaths in Sweden began falling (from a peak of about 100 per day) in mid-April 2020 to near-zero by late July, this decline was not quite as steep as elsewhere in Europe.[191] The overriding problem in Sweden, as in many countries, has been *the large number of deaths among people over 80, especially in long-term care facilities.*[30-32,191,195-197] The usual explanation for Sweden's death rate being higher than elsewhere in Scandinavia focuses instead on younger people continuing to congregate in bars and parks in Stockholm, the capital and hardest-hit part of the country,[3,191] who presumably then eventually infected older people (despite Swedes having much less inter-generational mixing compared to regions such as southern Europe). Yet by mid-May 2020, curiously only 7% of Stockholm residents had antibodies to the coronavirus[198] (half the percentage found, for example, in a rural part of Germany[159]). This is undoubtedly because many Swedes already lived alone, telecommuted, and as has happened elsewhere, had voluntarily adopted distancing and other prevention habits.

Furthermore, thanks to Sweden's generous immigration policies its non-European population is larger than in other Scandinavian countries, and has been disproportionately affected by Covid-19, purportedly due to a lack of culturally-tailored educational campaigns, a high prevalence of chronic health conditions, and crowded public housing.[197,199,200] Immigrants reportedly account for most deaths in Stockholm, notably including many Somalis,[197,200,201] who may be more vulnerable than other Africans due to civil wars having kept them from receiving the childhood tuberculosis vaccine,[202] which may offer partial protection against Covid-19.[203-205] Unlike elsewhere in Scandinavia, most of Stockholm's nursing home employees[199,200] (as well as many doctors and other medical professionals, who are said to have contributed substantially in the Covid-19 response) are non-

> Many Covid-19 prevention strategies have probably had little impact because they target potential risks accounting for only a small proportion of infections.

Europeans. Perhaps echoing difficult tradeoffs during the early AIDS years between wanting to avoid exacerbating homophobia and other persecution of marginalized groups while also needing to target prevention efforts for those at greatest risk, Swedish health authorities very understandably may be struggling to balance the need to more directly serve the communities suffering most from Covid-19, against the risk of inadvertently provoking a xenophobic backlash from increased attention to the immigrants' situation.[197,199,200]

It is noteworthy that some other countries such as Japan, with a low per-capita Covid-19 death rate despite having the world's oldest population, also never locked down.[206] And in the six midwestern and southern U.S. states that similarly did not fully shut down, as of early June 2020 observable increases in new cases had not occurred as compared to demographically similar rural states that implemented tight lockdowns.[207,208] A key conclusion from the experience of those various states and countries is not that death rates in such places have necessarily been *lower* than elsewhere, but rather if outcomes generally have not been *worse* this suggests that fairly similar results may be achievable at a less drastic economic – and quality-of-life – cost.[190] Of course, more urban regions will require different types and intensities of interventions than rural areas. As we ought to have learned from previous health crises including AIDS, the tendency to apply a one-size-fits-all approach should be reconsidered.[1,4,5,8] In any event, it is entirely conceivable that future medical historians will conclude that many current Covid-19 prevention strategies, including some that created substantial anxiety and hardship, probably had little impact because they targeted potential risks accounting for at most only a small proportion of total infections.[3,67,73,74]

12 LESSER KNOWN FACTS

■ **FACT 1:** The majority of infections have occurred within *clusters* of family members, coworkers, nursing home residents, prison inmates, and other persons in close and prolonged proximity.

"Clusters" of people living, working or otherwise spending *close* and *prolonged* time together,[69,209] especially in indoor settings with poor circulation and ventilation of air,[67,71,210-213] such as in certain factories, cruise ships, and churches, have been particularly affected by Covid-19. As previously discussed, long-term elderly care facilities have been extremely hard-hit.[30,31,160,196,197] In Canada, for example, 81% of all reported Covid-19 deaths were among elderly care residents, who account for only 1% of that country's population.[32] Meat and poultry plant workers are also especially vulnerable to infection because of working and living conditions common in the industry, including prolonged close contact among coworkers, typically cold and noisy indoor settings (often necessitating shouting to others), 8-12 hour shifts, group housing, and shared transportation.[214-216] Although farm workers work mainly outdoors, they also often share housing, group transportation, and other indoor exposures such as communal eating quarters.

A *JAMA* study reported that prisoners[217,218] were over five times more likely to become infected and three times more likely to die of Covid-19.[219] Mass transit, especially when people were crowded very closely together, undoubtedly was also a significant mode of transmission.[211] Perhaps not coincidentally, nearly all the places that experienced the largest Covid-19 outbreaks, including Wuhan, Milan, Madrid, London, and New York City, had heavily utilized mass transit systems (and often many smokers and worse air pollution, which may also be a factor[220]).

> Meat plant workers are vulnerable to infection due to prolonged close contact among coworkers, cold indoor settings, long shifts, and group housing.

- **FACT 2:** The admonition that people with Covid-19 symptoms or who test positive should remain home unless becoming very ill appears to have been a major driver of the pandemic.

Such public health pronouncements inadvertently but tragically led to a delay in seeking care, which diminished survival odds,[22,221] and also exposed household members to significant infection risk.[209-211] Contact tracing studies have identified the single largest source of infections as the sharing of living quarters.[209-211] Those Asian countries that quarantined infected persons *away* from home, in clinically provisioned camps or hotels, had much better success in controlling infections and, also importantly, in reducing death rates.[221] Iceland utilized a similarly successful approach, including use of a remote home quarantining method involving virtual medical supervision and counseling support.[222,223] It would seem that in most European countries and the U.S., where such crucial prevention measures, as well as rigorous tracing, largely have not been adopted, we instead have been grasping at much less important considerations. These include fixating on avoiding behaviors and settings where the actual risk is very low, such as fleeting public encounters, surface-based transmission, or beach visits.[3,27,71,73,74] Meanwhile, those measures which arguably could have the greatest prevention impact, such as reengineering buildings to improve air circulation (and possibly filtration), are still not widely prioritized.[213]

- **FACT 3:** Outdoor transmission is up to twenty times less likely than transmission indoors.

While perhaps the fact that outdoor transmission is less risky compared to being indoors is no longer particularly lesser-known, the huge differential in risk, which researchers have estimated to be 19 times lower, is worth noting.[212] This gigantic difference is due to various factors, including dissipation of droplets in the air (especially when windy) and the deactivating effects of ultraviolet radiation, in addition to heat and humidity.[224,225,226] Those investigators were from Japan, where the government has strongly urged the population to hold meetings and other events outdoors.[206] A contact tracing study in China found that 80% of infections involved house-

> Japanese investigators estimate being outdoors carries 19 times lower risk of infection than being indoors.

hold members and 34% involved mass transit (multiple possible transmission routes were assessed), whereas only *one* of the 7,324 infection events investigated was linked to casual outdoor transmission.[211]

Exercising or relaxing in parks or at the beach, even if momentarily getting close to other people – or joining in a mass protest march, especially if masks are commonly used – are not high-risk situations for spreading the virus.[3,27,71] In fact, now more than ever it is critically important for people of all ages to practice regular activity for physical[28,47,48,227] and mental health reasons.[43,44,227,228] Even indoor public exercise may be safe to resume, at least in low-prevalence settings and if precautions are taken. Preliminary findings from a large Norwegian trial found people who were randomized to work out at the gym did not have higher risk of acquiring the coronavirus compared to those randomized to remain home.[229]

■ **FACT 4:** *Voluntary* changes in behavior – widely adopted habits of routine hygiene, distancing, etc. – have been the main factor in slowing the pandemic.

Although governmental measures such as shelter-in-place orders undoubtedly saved lives, especially in densely populated areas such as Wuhan, New York, and Madrid, voluntary adoption of simple *behavioral changes* like routine hygiene practices and physical distancing have had the greatest impact.[3,207] Consistent with the experience of other public health challenges including HIV-AIDS, **coercive** measures such as issuing fines and arresting (or occasionally even shooting) people for violating lockdown and curfew orders, as has occurred in a number of places, have been much less effective in curbing the pandemic.[4,34,230-232] Many of the countries that had achieved the most successful responses, including South Korea, Hong Kong, Singapore, Japan, Taiwan, and Iceland, typically employed a more "surgical" or carefully targeted and evidence-based **public health** approach, focusing particularly on extensive testing, contact tracing, and quarantining.[3,25,176,206,222,223] As a result, they were also able – unlike countries that relied on a more "blunt

> Many successful countries have employed a carefully targeted **public health** approach, and were able to keep open large parts of the economy and society.

39

instrument" strategy of mandating total lockdowns – to keep open large parts of the economy and society, often including schools.

■ **FACT 5:** Despite the fear of health systems becoming overwhelmed, this has rarely occurred.

Although medical personnel in the hardest-hit areas have occasionally been stretched to the limit, thankfully health systems have generally not been massively overwhelmed, except briefly in a few places such as northern Italy and Madrid, and have been able to respond adequately (and often heroically). In New York City, for example, reportedly most of the 40,000 available ventilators were not utilized, and some makeshift temporary hospitals also went unused.[232] While flatten-the-curve emergency measures are part of the reason this occurred – and while at the time it certainly seemed better to be prepared than sorry – moving forward we now know this is unlikely to happen, especially in more rural areas. Many rural hospitals are now facing the *opposite* problem: recently so few patients have been admitted, in part because of ongoing fear of contracting the coronavirus, that many hospitals will probably end up going out of business.[233] A July 2020 analysis noted, "Thankfully, the scenario where hospitals across the country needed eight times their capacity did not happen. In the regions where the epidemic has already peaked, hospitals had sufficient capacity to care for all Covid-19 patients. On average, about one-third of hospital beds are available nationwide and most hospitals have plans for regional surges. Still, some cities or regions may have local surges that exceed hospital capacity, but this scenario should not be the norm."[234]

However, as the pandemic eventually expands into lower-income regions of the world including Africa and South Asia, the strain on already-fragile health systems will require ongoing attention and possibly international assistance.[36,184-89,235] Also, the situation in places like Houston and Arizona, where in late June and early July 2020 many intensive care units (ICUs) reached near-capacity levels, certainly merits careful evaluation.[236,237] Although the *proportion* of younger persons hospitalized with Covid-19 complications had increased, as would be expected since many more younger people were becoming infected, the absolute *numbers* of younger patients remained relatively low. Encouragingly, both the percentage of hospital patients requiring ICU care and the duration of hospitals stays have been declining significantly.[238,239]

- **FACT 6:** As devastating as this pandemic has been, it has killed almost as many people as the 1968-69 "Hong Kong Flu" pandemic.

Covid-19 has already killed almost as many persons as the approximately one million who succumbed globally to that also named "Forgotten Pandemic" (striking when the world's population was half of today's).[240] Especially if successful vaccines or more effective treatment regimes are not developed soon, the numbers of deaths will even end up surpassing the estimated 1.5 million who died from the "Asian Flu" pandemic of 1958. While the devastation already inflicted by Covid-19 should not be minimized, thankfully it is very unlikely to kill anywhere near the over 40 million persons (over 2 million in the U.S.) who die annually from largely preventable chronic conditions including diabetes, hypertension, obesity, and smoking.[241-243] In fact, these are the same underlying conditions that 1) disproportionately affect poor and minority populations, and 2) are associated with the vast majority of Covid-19 deaths.[59,60,61] *Prioritizing effective prevention of such chronic conditions could therefore also help reduce future severe illness and deaths from diseases such as Covid-19.*[3,62,63,65,243]

> Over 40 million die annually from largely preventable chronic conditions like diabetes, obesity, and smoking- the same predisposing conditions for dying from Covid-19.

- **FACT 7:** Many more people have died this year than usual from non-Covid-19 causes such as heart attack, stroke, and appendicitis because of being denied medical attention or due to avoiding hospitals out of fear of contracting the virus.

While probably most excess deaths (current mortality compared to death levels in previous years[192-194]) observed in various countries have resulted from the previously mentioned under-counting of official Covid-19 deaths, a substantial number were because of persons with other acute conditions who were turned away from hospitals, especially during the first months of the pandemic, due to an unrealized expectation of becoming overwhelmed by Covid-19 patients.[21,23] An even greater number of unnecessary deaths, which according to a July 2020 *JAMA* study have accounted for a third or more of excess mortality this year,[17,18] have occurred because of persons who, apparently from fear of acquiring the coronavirus, have avoided medical care for cardiac arrest, stroke, and other urgent non-Covid-19 conditions.[17,19-23] Some pregnant women (who appear somewhat more vulnerable to Covid-19-related complications, though not of death[244,245]) have also avoided giving birth in hospitals due to fear of contracting the disease.[22,246]

> A third of all excess deaths this year have been in persons who avoided urgent medical care from fear of Covid-19.

■ **FACT 8:** The media has tended to portray the more extreme aspects of the pandemic, feeding fear and anxiety.

Journalists deserve credit for drawing attention to the magnitude of this crisis, especially earlier on, as well as for meticulously investigating many complex aspects of the problem (hence the large number of informative news reports cited in the references below). In retrospect, however, along with many of us attempting to make sense of a complicated challenge, the media could have done some things better. The pervasive level of anxiety and fear surrounding this pandemic has been fed by stark mass media depictions of children dying from coronavirus-related causes or of young, healthy adults also succumbing. Although this sort of dramatic coverage may not involve fabrication of evidence, it tends to misrepresent the actual nature of the disease, skewing the public's perception toward believing that far more young and healthy people are being impacted than is in fact the case.

Furthermore, and perhaps reminiscent of "AIDS exceptionalism,"[9] the mass media typically does not contextualize the pain and loss caused by Covid-19. Without trivializing the pandemic's deadly impact, the public might be helped to place the disease into a broader perspective. In Texas, for example, as coronavirus cases continued escalating during the first week of July 2020, reported Covid-19 deaths averaged 42 per day[247] while average daily deaths from largely preventable heart disease in the state were about triple that amount.[248] (However, shortly thereafter Covid-19 deaths rose substantially for several weeks.) Some media coverage has reinforced other misperceptions, such as tending to focus on issues like crowded beaches as the presumed source of new infections and deaths,[27,71] rather than investigating much more important causes such as poor air circulation in buildings, shortages of nursing home employees, or the underlying reasons, including the obesity epidemic, for the high prevalence of preexisting chronic diseases.[31,62-64,160,213,243]

On the other hand, as during other health crises the media can play a useful role in educating the public. For example, a physician expert interviewed by NBC News in May 2020 patiently explained why there is no scientific reason, if precautions are taken, for grandparents to avoid spending time again with their grandchildren. As she creatively suggested to viewers, from a health perspective simple but important gestures such as allowing children to hug one's waist or being comfortable kissing the back of their heads is not risky. Even during periods of heightened concern triggered by surges in new cases, it is vital to not allow ourselves to fall into unnecessary anxiety or fear. Responsible media reporting could help greatly in this regard.

■ FACT 9: Some mitigation measures, particularly ventilators, have evidently done more harm than good.

While also not widely reported by the media, initial data suggested up to 85% of persons placed on ventilators for Covid-19 had died, although more recent evidence indicates such deaths have been substantially lower.[249,250] Certainly, doctors are learning to use improved strategies, including earlier provision of supplemental oxygen, and in countries like Germany have been encouraging people to seek treatment before symptoms become unbearable.[238,239,251]

■ FACT 10: The economic collapse and other outcomes of prolonged shutdowns have resulted in unprecedented consequences.

While in hindsight the motives behind the more severe lockdown measures may be understandable, it is evident they have also taken a huge economic and quality-of-life toll.[24,33-36,252] These repercussions have been *far more painfully experienced in socioeconomically disadvantaged communities*,[253] such as minority-owned businesses, for whom the long-term consequences appear dire.[254] And a May

2020 Kaiser Family Foundation analysis estimated that 27 million Americans had already lost their employer-based health insurance due to the economic downturn.[255,256] The harm of remaining inside often-cramped living quarters for extended durations must also be considered, including documented perilous upsurges in domestic violence,[37-39] child abuse,[40,41,146] obesity,[47,48] social isolation,[40,43,142] anxiety and depression,[43-45] automobile accident deaths,[257] and probably suicides.[45,258] According to a June 2020 analysis, drug overdoses in the U.S. shot up 42% during the previous month, after finally starting to decline just before the pandemic hit.[46] The stress of lockdowns is experienced even more intensely among people suffering from obsessive-compulsive disorder,[259,260] ADHD,[261] autism,[149] and other added challenges.

In poorer regions of the world such as Africa[185,188] and South Asia[23,262] (despite the perhaps still expanding epidemics in countries like India and South Africa), it is quite possible that the unintended repercussions from global lockdown measures could end up resulting in even more harm than good.[3,184,186,187,263] Indeed, in some places the harm done may eventually be of tragic proportions, including potentially vast increases in deaths due to hunger and malnutrition,[33,34,264] malaria,[265] tuberculosis,[266] measles,[267] AIDS,[268] and other diseases[269] – as vaccination,[267,270,271] maternal and child health care,[272,273] emergency food relief, HIV,[235] and other basic services are suspended due to lockdowns or deprioritized while efforts refocus on Covid-19.

Considering that young children are likely to be particularly impacted, this could represent an even greater magnitude of devastation if measured in terms of years-of-life lost rather than simply by counting excess deaths. Policy makers appear to be making enormously consequential decisions without fully considering some key demographic (and possibly significant climate[224-226] and/or childhood vaccine-related factors[203-205,274,275]) between lower-income

> In Africa and South Asia, the repercussions from lockdown measures may cause more harm than good.

tropical regions, characterized by more rural and much younger populations, and Europe and North America, with their more urban, considerably older and often more obese populations, which consequentially may have much greater vulnerability to Covid-19 mortality.[3,184-189]

- **FACT 11:** Even if a relatively effective vaccine is developed it may not be a perfect solution.

Based on experience with other respiratory pathogens and the emerging data on Covid-19, as discussed earlier most experts believe that previous infection from the novel coronavirus probably offers some degree of immunity, although it remains unclear exactly to what extent and especially for how long.[123,164,165,276] However, if prior exposure does *not* provide relatively long-lasting immunity, then vaccines are also very unlikely to work. Even if a successful vaccine is eventually developed, it may not be a perfect solution. While a relatively effective vaccine might be widely available by late 2020 at the earliest, as previously mentioned it could certainly take much longer.[178] Vaccines may be far less than 100% effective, especially if the virus mutates significantly, and regular booster shots and/or constant reformulation may be required, such as with annual flu shots.[123,164,165]

- **FACT 12:** There are however reasons to be hopeful we *can* return to (more) of a sense of "normality."

Intriguingly, there are suggestions that, at least in areas that were hard-hit, the coronavirus may becoming less *lethal*[277] (while evidently becoming more *contagious*[278]), a not uncommon pattern for viral parasites. Scientists in Italy, Spain, Israel, and the U.S. report discovering genetic mutations and other indications that the virus, through evolutionary self-selection, may be pursuing the kind of "don't burn the house" strategy that other pathogens regularly adopt in order not to kill too many of their hosts.[277] Although it may be premature to know whether this is actually taking place (which some other researchers dispute[279]), nevertheless it is curious that, while the number of daily new *cases* worldwide continued to climb steadily throughout the first half of 2020, from roughly late April through early June the daily average of reported Covid-19 *deaths* steadily declined, and then remained relatively flat through at least mid-July.[280]

Although this discrepancy is partly due to poor official recording of deaths as well as to greatly expanded testing, it may also relate to the fact that many recent infections have taken place in lower-income regions. Despite the worrisome vulnerability of weaker health care systems in such settings, the age pyramid is typically much more weighted toward younger people, who are of course far less likely to die from Covid-19.[184,185,187,189] There are increasingly clear indications of such a pattern occurring in India, for example.[281,282] However, time will tell whether global deaths continue to hover at around 5,000 a day or whether they might, following a U-shaped curve, begin once again to rise substantially.

A FEMA modeling study widely circulated in late April 2020 predicted that U.S. deaths would reach 3,000 per day by the end of May.[283] Thankfully, daily Covid-19 deaths actually continued falling in the U.S. (as in Europe) from around mid-April 2020, averaging less than 1,000 deaths per day between late May and late June, and then dropped even further through early July. Yet in late May reported *cases* began rising at an alarming rate, particularly in several southern and southwestern states and in southern California, areas that had largely evaded the initial wave earlier in the year. The reopening of bars, restaurants and other venues – more directly related to what can be termed "casual transmission" – is one reason for the surges in new cases.[284]

Nonetheless, it is likely that *most* recent infections are consistent with the predominant pattern so far throughout the world. As previously discussed, extensive contact tracing studies conducted in Wuhan, China in February 2020 and subsequent research in several other regions indicate that the large majority of coronavirus infections take place within *clusters* of family members, coworkers, inhabitants of Native American reservations, prisoners, and other persons spending prolonged periods of time in close proximity.[3,67,71,209-211] As the U.S. economy began to reopen in many states, it appears that workers in a variety of industries, especially lower-earning manual laborers, began getting exposed in far greater numbers.

> As the U.S. economy began reopening in many states, workers began getting exposed in far greater numbers.

The key question, of course, regards the magnitude of increased deaths that will inevitably follow the steep rise in reported *cases* in the southern and western parts of the U.S. The fact that starting in late June 2020 many ICUs reached or nearly reached capacity in places such as Houston is troubling.[236,237,239] Yet considering that the wave of infections had disproportionately struck younger people compared to the elderly, the eventual increase in deaths will likely be much less pronounced than during the crisis that befell parts of the East Coast, Midwest, and Europe earlier in 2020.[239,285] As of July 10, over a month after cases began increasing sharply in states including Texas, Florida, and California, the predicted jump in Covid-19 deaths had yet to materialize[286-288] (though deaths did eventually rise soon thereafter).

Given the soaring numbers of cases in June, the number of daily U.S. deaths eventually could even triple or more compared to the low point in early July of around 400 per day. Yet even in that unfortunate scenario, deaths are unlikely to rise anywhere nearly as sharply as had the tide of new cases. It may also be worth noting that if a sizeable portion of the population does end up becoming infected (perhaps due partly to the coronavirus having mutated over time to become more contagious[278]), while this may not necessarily approach herd immunity levels, as noted earlier substantially fewer people may therefore be at risk in a future wave(s). From a prevention perspective, a community where 30% have previously been infected is probably considerably less vulnerable than one where only 5% may have immunity.[123,179-181]

> A community where 30% of people have previously been infected is probably considerably less vulnerable than one where only 5% may have immunity.

In addition, research is *urgently needed regarding the prevalence, diagnosis, prognosis, and treatment options for longer-term Covid-19 complications,*[166-170] including post-traumatic stress disorder, which may be fairly common.[289,290] Another crucial concern – in addition to the often-mishandled political leadership in the U.S., Brazil,[291,292] the U.K., Iran, etc. – is the much higher Covid-19 death rate in African-American communities, due among other reasons to a greater prevalence of predisposing conditions such as diabetes, obesity, and hypertension.[59,62,243] At the same time, the rise in Covid-19 cases in many states including Texas, Florida, Arizona, and California have disproportionately occurred not only in much younger persons but particularly among Latinos, including many undocumented immigrants with little if any access to health care.[293,294,295] Members of these communities tend to work in higher-risk occupations such as meatpacking plants, to share more crowded living quarters, and otherwise are often less able to practice distancing and other prevention measures. Additionally, Latino cultures tend to be, fairly similarly to southern Europeans, more physically demonstrative.

As of mid-June 2020, 46% of cases in North Carolina were reported among Hispanics, who make up just 9% of the state's population.[296] Interestingly, only 8% of recorded Covid-19 deaths occurred among this population (though likely due in part to under-reporting issues), compared to 33% of deaths taking place among African-Americans, who comprise 22% of the state's residents. In California, 57% of reported cases have been among Latinos, and the CDC estimated that by late June 2020 33% of all cases nationally had occurred in Latinos, about double their proportion of the U.S. population.[293,297]

In Arizona, where in early July 2020 per-capita cases soared the most of any state, according to the 2010 Census 30% of the population were Latinos, and data from June 2020 indicate the per-capita number of Covid-19 cases among Latinos was more than twice as high as other ethnic groups in the state.[298] On July 7, 2020 the CDC reported on data from workers in 329 U.S. meat and poultry facilities across 23 states, finding that 56% of cases had occurred among Hispanic employees, who made up just 30% of the workers.[215,216] Perhaps paralleling the Swedish dilemma mentioned earlier, some regional health authorities may feel torn between the need to focus where, epidemiologically, the problem is centered yet they may also be hesitant, especially given the politically explosive issue of immigration, about drawing attention to the fact that Latino communities are being overwhelmingly affected.

....

Many had worried that the mass street rallies over George Floyd's murder carried out in many places including Minneapolis, Seattle, Washington, D.C., and New York City would result in spikes of new Covid-19 cases. Yet several months later no notable increases in these regions had been observed, and routine testing of many thousands of protestors in those cities yielded seropositivity rates of about 1%, lower than in the surrounding communities.[299-301] (Previously, it had been incorrectly predicted that anti-lockdown protests in places like Michigan would similarly stoke the epidemic.) Future historians may view this as a pivotal moment when a key segment of the U.S. population not only took to the streets to protest police brutality and racism, but as a result also began to regain a meaningful sense of public "normality" for the first time since the pandemic crisis began. (Following the subsequent upsurge in Covid-19 cases in several parts of the U.S., this palpable shift in mood sadly was short-lived, as starkly borne out in July 2020 polling data.[302])

Several months after the Floyd street protests, associated increases in Covid-19 cases had evidently not occurred.

However, given that deaths appear to be declining over time (certainly in proportion to the numbers of new cases), along with the prospect of vaccines on the horizon, researchers and clinicians are also hopeful because a slew of medications and procedures to reduce the risk of severe illness and death are being developed and tested, in addition to rapid and affordable home tests. Such drugs include antiviral combinations and the anti-inflammatory steroid dexamethasone, as well as the possibility that ongoing trials of century-old childhood vaccines against tuberculosis and polio may provide some protection against the new coronavirus.[203-205]

Although certainly much pain and death still lies ahead, these developments along with improved clinical practices, which are clearly another reason for the mortality decline,[238,239,249,250] offer some hope that the overall situation may turn around before much longer. Despite the potential for a larger wave in late 2020, perhaps including in some places that were hit hard earlier on, both the public and scientists know much more about this virus than we did just a few months earlier. And if another big wave does eventually materialize, we will be better prepared and hopefully smarter about focusing our energies on using the most effective prevention measures.

CONCLUSION

This review of the existing (and certainly often-changing) evidence has attempted to synthesize and present the best available data – and apparent myths – regarding the novel coronavirus and the global pandemic it has unleashed. All of us understandably are fearful or at least seriously concerned. (As I write these final words my teenage daughters, who just boarded a plane to visit me, are texting anxiously because the flight is full and someone's sitting in the same row.) Yet I hope that a careful examination of the scientific evidence has provided some practical suggestions for lowering the risk of illness and death and helped to alleviate anxiety and fear. I have been reassuring my normally adventurous elderly mother in California and my previously energetic mother-in-law in Madrid that they can, and indeed should, resume enjoying daily walks and (with care) socializing. And I have advised my sister, who has recovered from Covid-19, that very likely she is immune to re-infection, at least for the near-to-medium future.

However, it is of immediate concern that the peak in cases may not quite have been reached yet in some areas, including parts of Latin America,[303] South Asia,[23,262] and Africa.[304] Although things remain painful and scary, and while understandably there is hesitation to let down our guard (and regardless of whatever ideological controversy may be broiling at the moment), it is imperative to remember that spikes and occasionally outright waves of cases are inevitable nearly everywhere. And as testing continues to increase, more cases will invariably be found. In fact, we must continue expanding testing services to allow for early identification of cases, following those up with contact tracing, and ideally, despite seemingly immense logistical and cultural challenges, when possible quarantining new cases away from home. Yet the level of deaths must always be the most important indicator to monitor. We need to strategically prioritize how best to prevent severe (including longer-term) illness and **deaths**, instead of focusing overwhelmingly on attempting to eliminate new **cases**.

> We must strategically prioritize how best to prevent severe illness and **deaths** rather than our overwhelming focus on eliminating new **cases**

On a more reflective note, while the previous respiratory pandemics of 1918-1919,

1958, and 1968-69 killed a horrifying number of people, in an evolutionary sense they also acted like enormous global vaccines: subsequent generations have to a large degree been naturally immunized from the three major influenza strains introduced by those huge pandemics.[305] It is quite plausible that the four known older strains of coronaviruses – which today cause many of the common colds that children and others acquire but are only rarely killed by – long ago made their entrance as similarly murderous pandemics.

Of course, we must continue doing everything possible to develop effective vaccines, medications, and other useful mitigation approaches. We must also attempt to prevent the next deadly – and potentially even more horrific – pandemic, such as through banning international traffic in exotic animals like pangolins, which may have served as an intermediary species to introduce a bat coronavirus into human beings.[306,307] In addition, we might conceivably try viewing Covid-19 not only as an enemy to be defeated but, from a longer-term and more ecological perspective, as a part of the natural world with which our species must, painfully but out of necessity, learn somehow to co-exist. If this virus is indeed on an evolutionary trajectory toward advancing its survivability through becoming more contagious and less deadly over time,[277,278] in the future it may eventually join its four cousins to become the newest widely circulating but uncommonly fatal coronavirus.

A May 2020 *Atlantic* essay advised it is time to figure out, as we have done with other health challenges such as AIDS, "how to have a (safer) life during a pandemic."[8] As an epidemiologist, teacher, son, and father myself, I agree it is time to move beyond excessive anxiety and fear. While carefully evaluating the best ways to practice precautions, we may also learn how to *live* better, grateful for what joy we can experience despite the challenging circumstances this novel virus has thrust upon us all.

ACKNOWLEDGMENTS

This book could not have been completed without the amazing brainstorming, editing, and other kind assistance of Coloma Araujo, Jeffrey Ashley, Glenn Post, David Wolfson, Steve Hodgins, and Mark Tilton. The following persons also generously contributed to the formulation, refinement, and editing: Robert Bailey, Norman Hearst, Roy Jacobstein, Ariel Halperin, Leila Halperin, Lee Ross, Arthur Allen, Helen Jackson, David Alnwick, Patricia Rice Doran, Rick Gore, Ben Cox, Matt Irwin, Joshua Sharfstein, Kate Crawford, Robert Norton, Juan Davalos, Richard Wamai, Soren Geiger, Jamie Tipton, and Jim Shelton. Cover art and layout assistance by Maribel Liberal and Ferenc Rozumberski.

Author can be contacted at: **dhalpe@ad.unc.edu** *and* **@daniel_halperin**

ABOUT THE AUTHOR

Daniel Halperin, Ph.D. is Adjunct (Full) Professor at the University of North Carolina Gillings School of Global Public Health in Chapel Hill. He has conducted epidemiological and anthropological research for over forty years in Latin America, sub-Saharan Africa and other regions, and previously taught at Harvard School of Public Health, the University of California at Berkeley, and the Ponce School of Medicine in Puerto Rico. He served over five years as Senior HIV Prevention Advisor at the US Agency for International Development (USAID). Dr. Halperin co-authored a *New York Times* "Editor's Choice" book on the AIDS pandemic and has published over 60 peer-reviewed articles on infectious diseases in leading scientific journals, as well as a number of opinion pieces in the *Washington Post, New York Times, Financial Times,* and elsewhere.

REFERENCES

Note regarding cited references: Whenever possible, peer-reviewed articles and books (or if unavailable, papers from the "gray" literature) are cited. As unfortunately there remains a shortage of academic publications on this topic, many of the citations below are drawn from the popular press (often written by scientists or containing data from interviews with researchers, etc.).

1. Halperin DT, Steiner M, Cassell M, et al. [149 signers in total]. The time has come for common ground on preventing sexual transmission of HIV. *Lancet.* 2004;364 (9449):1913-15. **https://pubmed.ncbi.nlm.nih.gov/15566989/**

2. *Glob Health Sci Pract.* Baltimore: Johns Hopkins Univ. **https://www.ghspjournal.org/**

3. Halperin DT. Coping with COVID-19: learning from past pandemics to avoid pitfalls and panic. *Glob Health Sci Pract.* 2020;8(2). **https://doi.org/10.9745/GHSP-D-20-00189 https://www.ghspjournal.org/content/8/2/155**

4. Timberg C, Halperin D. Tinderbox: How the West Sparked the AIDS Epidemic and How the World Can Finally Overcome It. N. York: Penguin Books; 2012. **www.tinderboxbook.com**

5. Potts M, Halperin DT, Kirby D, et al. Reassessing HIV prevention. *Science.* 2008;320 (5877):749–750. **https://science.sciencemag.org/content/320/5877/749.full**

6. Pereira C. How HIV/AIDS changed the world. *Economist.* June 25, 2020. **https://www.economist.com/books-and-arts/2020/06/25/how-hiv-aids-changed-the-world**

7. Roiphe K. Last Night in Paradise: Sex and Morals at the Century's End. New York: Little, Brown & Co.; 1997.

8. Marcus J. Quarantine fatigue is real. *The Atlantic.* May 11, 2020. **https://www.theatlantic.com/ideas/archive/2020/05/quarantine-fatigue-real-and-shaming-people-wont-help/611482/**

9. Halperin D. Putting a plague in perspective. *New York Times.* January 1, 2008. **https://www.nytimes.com/2008/01/01/opinion/01halperin.html**

10. Zakaria, F. The pandemic is too important to be left to the scientists. *Washington Post.* April 30, 2020. **https://www.washingtonpost.com/opinions/itll-take-more-than-just-scientists-to-stem-this-pandemic/2020/04/30/9ee1daf6-8b1d-11ea-9dfd-990f9dcc71fc_story.html?itid=ap_fareedzakaria**

11. Russell S. Circumcision may be potent AIDS weapon. Studies reveal pattern in African epidemic. *SF Chronicle.* July 11, 2000. **https://www.sfgate.com/health/article/Circumcision-May-Be-Potent-AIDS-Weapon-Studies-3304032.php**

12. Timberg C. Death counts become the rhythm of the pandemic in the absence of national mourning. *Washington Post.* May 24, 2020. **https://www.washingtonpost.com/technology/2020/05/24/death-counts-become-rhythm-pandemic-absence-national-mourning/**

13. Witte M, Allen M. A meta-analysis of fear appeals: implications for effective public health campaigns. *Health Educ Behav*. 2000; 27(5):591–615. **https://journals.sagepub.com/doi/abs/10.1177/109019810002700506**

14. Stephens B. It's dangerous to be ruled by fear. *New York Times*. March 20, 2020. **https://www.nytimes.com/2020/03/20/opinion/coronavirus-data.html**

15. Marsh A. How we can keep fear from spiraling out of our control. *Washington Post*. June 23, 2020. **https://www.washingtonpost.com/opinions/2020/06/23/era-covid-19-our-fear-doesnt-have-define-us/?arc404=true**

16. Ripley A. Five ways to conquer your Covid-19 fears. *Washington Post*. April 6, 2020. **https://washingtonpost.com/opinions/2020/04/06/five-ways-conquer-your-covid-19-fears/**

17. Thebault R, Bernstein L, Tran AB, Shin Y. Heart conditions drove spike in deaths beyond those attributed to Covid-19, analysis shows. Fear of seeking care in hospitals overwhelmed by the pandemic may have caused thousands of deaths, experts say. *Washington Post*. July 2, 2020. **https://www.washingtonpost.com/graphics/2020/investigations/coronavirus-excess-deaths-heart/**

18. Woolf SH, Chapman DA, Sabo RT, Weinberger DM, Hill L. Excess deaths from COVID-19 and other causes, March-April 2020. *JAMA*. 2020. doi:10.1001/jama.2020.11787. **https://jamanetwork.com/journals/jama/fullarticle/2768086**

19. Lu D. There has been an increase in other causes of deaths, not just coronavirus. *New York Times*. June 1, 2020; **https://www.nytimes.com/interactive/2020/06/01/us/coronavirus-deaths-new-york-new-jersey.html**

20. Hafner K. Fear of Covid-19 leads other patients to decline critical treatment. Psychologists say anxiety and uncertainty prompt irrational decisions — like turning down a transplant when an organ becomes available. *NY Times*. May 25, 2020. **https://www.nytimes.com/2020/05/25/health/coronavirus-cancer-heart-treatment.html?referringSource=articleShare**

21. Bernstein B, Sellers FS. Patients with heart attacks, strokes and even appendicitis vanish from hospitals. *Washington Post*. April 19, 2020. **https://www.washingtonpost.com/health/patients-with-heart-attacks-strokes-and-even-appendicitis-vanish-from-hospitals/2020/04/19/9ca3ef24-7eb4-11ea-9040-68981f488eed_story.html**

22. Rao A. 'People are dying at home': virus fears deter seriously ill from hospitals. *Guardian*. May 6, 2020. **https://www.theguardian.com/world/2020/may/06/dying-at-home-non-covid-19-hospitals-coronavirus**

23. Kendrick M. COVID. 'with' 'of' or 'because of'. *Malcolmkendrick.org blog*. April 6, 2020. **https://drmalcolmkendrick.org/2020/04/06/covid-with-of-or-because-of/**

24. Friedman TL. A plan to get America back to work. *New York Times*. March 22, 2020. **https://www.nytimes.com/2020/03/22/opinion/coronavirus-economy.html**

25. Leung G. Lockdown can't last forever: here's how to lift it. *New York Times*. April 6, 2020. **https://www.nytimes.com/2020/04/06/opinion/coronavirus-end-social-distancing.html**

26. Walsh B. The U.S. divide on coronavirus masks. *Axios*. June 24, 2020. **https://www.axios.com/political-divide-coronavirus-masks-1053d5bd-deb3-4cf4-9570-0ba492134f3e.html**

27.	Tufekci Z. Scolding beachgoers isn't helping. People complain that going to the shore is a careless act during a pandemic, but the science so far suggests otherwise. *Atlantic.* July 4, 2020. **https://www.theatlantic.com/health/archive/2020/07/it-okay-go-beach/613849/**

28.	Miller AM. Stop shaming people for going outside. The risks are generally low, and the benefits are endless. *Business Insider.* April 25, 2020. **https://www.businessinsider.com/you-can-still-go-outsidewhile-quarantining-sheltering-in-place-2020-4**

29.	Cowburn A. Coronavirus: quarantine policy for travelers 'completely useless', says scientist who co-discovered Ebola. *The Independent.* June 21, 2020. **https://www.independent.co.uk/news/uk/politics/peter-piot-ebola-coronavirus-quarantine-boris-johnson-a9577786.html**

30.	Roy A. 43% of COVID-19 deaths are in nursing homes and assisted living facilities housing 0.6% of U.S. *Forbes.* May 26, 2020. **https://www.forbes.com/sites/theapothecary/2020/05/26/nursing-homes-assisted-living-facilities-0-6-of-the-u-s-population-43-of-u-s-covid-19-deaths/#5e4a270174cd**

31.	Whoriskey P, Cenziper D. Hundreds of nursing homes ran short on staff, protective gear as more than 30,000 residents died during pandemic. *Washington Post.* June 4, 2020. **https://www.washingtonpost.com/business/2020/06/04/nursing-homes-coronavirus-deaths/**

32.	Coletta, A. Canada's nursing home crisis: 81 percent of coronavirus deaths are in long-term care facilities. *Washington Post.* May 18, 2020. **https://www.washingtonpost.com/world/the_americas/coronavirus-canada-long-term-care-nursing-homes/2020/05/18/01494ad4-947f-11ea-87a3-22d324235636_story.html**

33.	Hohmann J, Alfaro M. Billions are out of work and millions of kids could die from coronavirus's economic fallout. *Washington Post.* May 15, 2020. **https://www.washingtonpost.com/news/powerpost/paloma/daily-202/2020/05/15/daily-202-billions-are-out-of-work-and-millions-of-kids-could-die-from-coronavirus-s-economic-fallout/5ebe2696602ff11bb1182c6d/**

34.	Abi-Habib M, Yasir S. India's coronavirus lockdown leaves vast numbers stranded and hungry. *New York Times.* March 29, 2020. **https://www.nytimes.com/2020/03/29/world/asia/coronavirus-india-migrants.html**

35.	Coronavirus: worst economic crisis since 1930s depression, IMF says. *BBC News.* April 9, 2020. **https://www.bbc.com/news/business-52236936**

36.	Covid-19 is undoing years of progress in curbing global poverty. *Economist.* May 23, 2020. **https://www.economist.com/international/2020/05/23/covid-19-is-undoing-years-of-progress-in-curbing-global-poverty**

37.	Bettinger-Lopez C, Bro A. *A Double Pandemic: Domestic Violence in the Age of COVID-19.* Council on Foreign Relations Brief. May 13, 2020. **https://www.cfr.org/in-brief/double-pandemic-domestic-violence-age-covid-19**

38.	Bosman J. Domestic violence calls mount as restrictions linger: 'no one can leave'. *New York Times.* May 15, 2020. **https://www.nytimes.com/2020/05/15/us/domestic-violence-coronavirus.html**

39.	Zakaria R. Domestic violence and coronavirus: hell behind closed doors. *The Nation.* April 2, 2020. **https://www.thenation.com/article/society/domestic-violence-coronavirus/**

40. Jagannathan M. How the stress and isolation of coronavirus could create "a perfect storm" for child abuse and neglect — and what you can do to help. *Market Watch*. May 7, 2020. **https://www.marketwatch.com/story/how-the-stress-and-isolation-of-coronavirus-could-create-a-perfect-storm-for-child-abuse-and-neglect-and-what-you-can-do-to-help-2020-05-06**

41. Woodall C. As hospitals see more severe child abuse injuries during coronavirus, "the worst is yet to come." *USA Today*. May 13, 2020. **https://www.usatoday.com/story/news/nation/2020/05/13/hospitals-seeing-more-severe-child-abuse-injuries-during-coronavirus/3116395001/**

42. Hayden S. 'There is violence in the house': children living under lockdown risk abuse the world over. *Telegraph*. June 3, 2020. **https://www.telegraph.co.uk/global-health/science-and-disease/violence-house-children-living-africas-strictest-lockdown-risk/**

43. Morrison N. It's not children's education we should worry about, it's their mental health. *Forbes*. May 15, 2020. **https://www.forbes.com/sites/nickmorrison/2020/05/15/its-not-childrens-education-we-should-worry-about-its-their-mental-health/#5bf84951fcbb**

44. Fowers A, Wan W. A third of Americans now show signs of clinical anxiety or depression, Census Bureau finds amid coronavirus pandemic. *Washington Post*. May 26, 2020. **https://www.washingtonpost.com/health/2020/05/26/americans-with-depression-anxiety-pandemic/?arc404=true**

45. Lardieri A. Coronavirus pandemic causing anxiety, depression in Americans, CDC finds. The CDC survey found that essential workers and young people have been more mentally affected by the pandemic. *US News and World Reports*. August 13, 2020. **https://www.usnews.com/news/health-news/articles/2020-08-13/coronavirus-pandemic-causing-anxiety-depression-in-americans-cdc-finds**

46. Wan W, Long H. 'Cries for help': Drug overdoses are soaring during the coronavirus pandemic. Suspected overdoses nationally jumped 18 percent in March, 29 percent in April and 42 percent in May, data from ambulance teams, hospitals and police shows. *Washington Post*. July 1, 2020. **https://www.washingtonpost.com/health/2020/07/01/coronavirus-drug-overdose/**

47. Rundle AG, Park Y, Herbstman JB, Kinsey EW, Wang YC. COVID-19 related school closings and risk of weight gain among children. *Obesity*. 2020;28(6):1008–1009. **https://onlinelibrary.wiley.com/doi/full/10.1002/oby.22813**

48. McNiff S. Lockdowns making things worse for obese Americans. *WebMD*. June 15, 2020. **https://www.webmd.com/lung/news/20200615/lockdowns-making-things-worse-for-obese-americans#1**

49. Chaker AM. The strain the covid pandemic is putting on marriages. Coronavirus stress has produced a pressure cooker inside homes, hurting even strong partnerships and, experts say, likely breaking others. *Wall Street Journal*. August 4, 2020. **https://www.wsj.com/articles/the-strain-the-covid-pandemic-is-putting-on-marriages-11596551839**

50. Sullum J. Do the divergent results of COVID-19 antibody studies reflect real differences? *Reason*. May 18, 2020. **https://reason.com/2020/05/18/do-the-divergent-results-of-covid-19-antibody-studies-reflect-real-differences/**

51. Cunningham PW. Why determining the coronavirus death rate is so tricky. *Washington Post*. July 10, 2020. **https://www.washingtonpost.com/news/powerpost/paloma/the-health-202/2020/07/10/thehealth-202-why-determining-the-coronavirus-death-rate-is-so-tricky/5f0727f088e0fa7b44f711fd/**

52. McNeil DG. The pandemic's big mystery: how deadly is the coronavirus? Even with more than 500,000 dead worldwide, scientists are struggling to learn how often the virus kills. *New York Times.* July 4, 2020. **https://www.nytimes.com/2020/07/04/health/coronavirus-death-rate.html**

53. Richardson I. Fact check: CDC's estimates COVID-19 death rate around 0.26%, doesn't confirm it. *USA Today.* June 5, 2020. **https://www.usatoday.com/story/news/factcheck/2020/06/05/fact-checkcdc-estimates-covid-19-death-rate-0-26/5269331002/**

54. Spiegelhalter D. What have been the fatal risks of Covid, particularly to children and younger adults? University of Cambridge, Winton Centre for Risk and Evidence Communication. June 13, 2020. **https://medium.com/wintoncentre/what-have-been-the-fatal-risks-of-covid-particularly-to-children-and-younger-adults-a5cbf7060c49**

55. Rettner R. How does the new coronavirus compare with the flu? *Live Science.* May 14, 2020. **https://www.livescience.com/new-coronavirus-compare-with-flu.html**

56. Gagnon A, Miller MS, Hallman SA, et al. Age-specific mortality during the 1918 influenza pandemic: unravelling the mystery of high young adult mortality. *PLoS One.* 2013;8(8):e69586. **https://www.ncbi.nlm.nih.gov/pmc/articles/PMC3734171/**

57. Spanish flu: the deadliest pandemic in history. *Live Science.* March 12, 2020. **https://www.livescience.com/spanish-flu.html**

58. The Covid age penalty: new patient data offers a guide to opening while protecting seniors. *Wall St J.* June 12, 2020. **https://www.wsj.com/articles/the-covid-age-penalty-11592003287**

59. Garg S, Kim K, Whitaker M. Hospitalization rates and characteristics of patients hospitalized with laboratory-confirmed coronavirus disease 2019-COVID-NET, 14 states, March 1-30, 2020. *Morb Mortal Wkly Rep.* 2020; 69(15);458–464. **https://www.cdc.gov/mmwr/volumes/69/wr/mm6915e3.htm**

60. Ebhardt T, Remondini C, Bertacche M. 99% of those who died from virus had other illness, Italy says. *Bloomberg News.* March 18, 2020. **https://www.bloomberg.com/news/articles/2020-03-18/99-of-those-who-died-from-virus-had-other-illness-italy-says**

61. World Health Organization (WHO). *Report of the WHO-China Joint Mission on Coronavirus Disease 2019 (COVID-19).* **https://www.who.int/docs/default-source/coronaviruse/who-china-joint-mission-on-covid-19-final-report.pdf**

62. Forrest A. Coronavirus: obesity doubles risk of needing hospital treatment, study suggests. *The Independent.* May 7, 2020. **https://www.independent.co.uk/news/health/coronavirus-obesity-doubles-risk-hospital-treatment-covid-19-a9503196.html**

63. Rollet J. Obesity triples odds of more severe symptoms with COVID-19. *Healio.* May 20, 2020. **https://www.healio.com/news/endocrinology/20200520/obesity-triples-odds-of-more-severe-symptoms-with-Covid-19**

64. Popkin B, Du S, Green WD, et al. Individuals with obesity and COVID-19: a global perspective on the epidemiology and biological relationships. *Obesity Reviews.* 2020. **https://onlinelibrary.wiley.com/doi/full/10.1111/obr.13128**

65. Patanavanich R, Glantz SA. Smoking is associated with COVID-19 progression: a meta-analysis. *MedRxiv.* 2020; **https://doi.org/10.1101/2020.04.13.20063669**

66. Van Zyl-Smit RN, Richards G, Leone FT. Tobacco smoking and COVID-19 infection. *The Lancet Respiratory Med.* 2020; DOI: **https://doi.org/10.1016/S2213-2600(20)30239-3**.

67. Bromage E. The risks: know them, avoid them. *Erin Bromage: COVID-19 Musings blog.* May 6, 2020. **https://erinbromage.wixsite.com/Covid-19/post/the-risks-know-them-avoid-them**

68. Camero K. How long you are exposed to coronavirus can determine if you get sick, experts say. *Miami Herald.* May 19, 2020. **https://www.miamiherald.com/news/coronavirus/article242846836.html**

69. Hernandez D, Toy S, McKay B. How exactly do you catch Covid-19? There is a growing consensus. *Wall St. J.* June 16, 2020. **https://www.wsj.com/articles/how-exactly-do-you-catch-covid-19-there-is-a-growing-consensus-11592317650**

70. Kayat S. Does a high viral load make coronavirus worse? A high prevalence of particles makes patients more infectious, but it is unclear if it leads to a more severe infection. *Aljazeera.* May 29, 2020. **https://www.aljazeera.com/indepth/features/doctor-note-high-viral-load-coronavirus-worse-200515075609542.html**

71. Amid confusion about reopening, an expert explains how to assess COVID-19 risk. *NPR.* June 17, 2020. **https://www.npr.org/2020/06/17/879255417/amid-confusion-about-reopening-an-expert-explains-how-to-assess-covid-risk**

72. Goldman E. Exaggerated risk of transmission of COVID-19 by fomites. *Lancet Infect Dis.* 2020. https://doi.org/10.1016/S1473-3099(20)30561-2 **https://www.thelancet.com/action/showPdf?pii=S1473-3099(20)30561-2**

73. Jones AM. Expert says studies on risk of virus transmission through surfaces don't reflect real world. *CTV News.* July 7, 2020. **https://www.ctvnews.ca/health/coronavirus/expert-says-studies-on-risk-ofvirus-transmission-through-surfaces-don-t-reflect-real-world-1.5015069**

74. Miller A, Pelley L. Why it may be harder to catch COVID-19 from surfaces than we first thought. Lack of evidence for infection from surfaces raises doubts about transmission. *CBC News.* July 11, 2020. **https://www.cbc.ca/news/health/coronavirus-surfaces-groceries-packages-playgrounds-1.5645602**

75. Kluger J. As disinfectant use soars to fight Coronavirus, so do accidental poisonings. *Time.* April 20, 2020. **https://time.com/5824316/coronavirus-disinfectant-poisoning/**

76. Cleaning and Disinfection for Households: Interim Recommendations for U.S. Households with Suspected or Confirmed Coronavirus Disease 2019 (COVID-19). 2020; Atlanta: CDC. **https://www.cdc.gov/coronavirus/2019-ncov/prevent-getting-sick/cleaning-disinfection.html**

77. Why you shouldn't wear gloves to the grocery store. Wearing gloves doesn't give you perfect protection against COVID-19. *Cleveland Clinic.* April 15, 2020. **https://health.clevelandclinic.org/why-you-shouldnt-wear-gloves-to-the-grocery-store/**

78. Gallagher S. Coronavirus: can latex gloves protect you from catching deadly virus? *The Independent.* May 29, 2020. **https://www.independent.co.uk/life-style/health-and-families/coronavirus-do-gloveswork-stop-virus-spread-symptoms-outbreak-a9362871.html**

79. *FDA Advises Consumers Not to Use Hand Sanitizer Products Manufactured by Eskbiochem.* FDA. 2020; **https://www.fda.gov/news-events/press-announcements/coronavirus-covid-19-update-fda-takes-action-warn-protect-consumers-dangerous-alcohol-based-hand**

80. Buchwald E. Americans are stocking up on disinfectant wipes, but will they kill coronavirus? *Market Watch*. March 9, 2020. **https://www.marketwatch.com/story/americans-are-stocking-up-on-disinfectant-wipes-but-will-they-kill-this-coronavirus-2020-03-05**

81. Bhargava HD. Mistakes you're making with antibacterial wipes. *WebMD*. June 25, 2020. **https://www.webmd.com/cold-and-flu/ss/slideshow-mistakes-antibacterial-wipes?ecd=wnl_spr_070920&ctr=wnl-spr-070920_nsl-LeadModule_cta&mb=OwCxcQ2sCvvWcxMEQZbEF3g0WleHxvlqvmtkKkloyeM%3d**

82. Lee B. For COVID-19 coronavirus, how well do thermometer guns even work? *Forbes*. February 16, 2020. **https://www.forbes.com/sites/brucelee/2020/02/16/for-covad-19-coronavirus-how-well-do-thermometer-guns-even-work/#8a9f96d2af91**

83. Li YY, Wang JX, Chen X. Can a toilet promote virus transmission? From a fluid dynamics perspective. *Physics of Fluids*. 2020;32(6); **doi.org/10.1063/5.0013318.**

84. Could 'toilet plumes' spread the new coronavirus? *Advisory Board*. June 23, 2020. **https://www.advisory.com/daily-briefing/2020/06/24/toilet-plumes**

85. Mandavilli A. 239 experts with one big claim: the coronavirus is airborne. The W.H.O. has resisted mounting evidence that viral particles floating indoors are infectious, some scientists say. The agency maintains the research is still inconclusive. *New York Times*. July 4, 2020. **https://www.nytimes.com/2020/07/04/health/239-experts-with-one-big-claim-the-coronavirus-is-airborne.html**

86. Gorski D. Is COVID-19 transmitted by airborne aerosols? A recurring debate about COVID-19 bubbled up late last week, when a group of scientists announced an as-yet unpublished open letter to the World Health Organization arguing that COVID-19 transmission is airborne and urging it to change its recommendations. What is this debate about, and, if coronavirus is airborne, should we be more scared? *Science-Based Medicine*. July 6, 2020. **https://sciencebasedmedicine.org/is-covid-19-transmitted-by-airborne-aerosols**

87. Odds of catching COVID-19 on an airplane are slimmer than you think, scientists say. *CNN Wire*. August 23, 2020. **https://abc7chicago.com/plane-air-travel-covid-odds/6382471/**

88. *Coronavirus Disease 2019 (COVID-19) Situation Report-73*. Geneva: WHO. April 2, 2020. **https://www.who.int/docs/default-source/coronaviruse/situation-reports/20200402-sitrep-73-covid-19.pdf?sfvrsn=5ae25bc7_2**

89. Furukawa NW, Brooks JT, Sobel J. Evidence supporting transmission of severe acute respiratory syndrome coronavirus 2 while presymptomatic or asymptomatic. *Emerg Infect Dis*. 2020; **https://doi.org/10.3201/eid2607.201595.**

90. Sax P. What we know – and what we don't – about 'asymptomatic COVID-19'. *WBUR*. June 26, 2020. **https://www.wbur.org/commonhealth/2020/06/26/asymptomatic-covid-faq-what-we-know**

91. Howard J. Coronavirus spread by asymptomatic people 'appears to be rare,' WHO official says. *CNN*. June 9, 2020. **https://www.cnn.com/2020/06/08/health/coronavirus-asymptomatic-spread-who-bn/index.html**

92. Oran DP, Topol EJ. Prevalence of asymptomatic SARS-CoV-2 infection: a narrative review. *Ann Intern Med*. 2020. doi:10.7326/M20-3012. (*See June 10, 2020 online Comment: Halperin DT, "A very useful, also highly problematic review article."*) **https://www.acpjournals.org/doi/10.7326/M20-3012**

93. Kucirka LM, Lauer SA, Laeyendecker O, Boon D, Lessler J. Variation in false-negative rate of reverse transcriptase polymerase chain reaction-based SARS-CoV-2 tests by time since exposure. *Ann Intern Med* 2020;May 13:[Epub ahead of print]. **https://www.ncbi.nlm.nih.gov/pmc/articles/PMC7240870/**

94. Wei WE, Li Z, Chiew CJ, Yong SE, Toh MP, Lee VJ. Presymptomatic transmission of SARS-CoV-2 – Singapore, January 23-March 16, 2020. *MMWR Morb Mortal Wkly Rep.* 2020;69:411–415. DOI: **https://www.cdc.gov/mmwr/volumes/69/wr/mm6914e1.htm**

95. Arons MM, Hatfield KM, Reddy SC, et al. Presymptomatic SARS-CoV-2 infections and transmission in a skilled nursing facility. *N Engl J Med.* 2020; 382:2081-2090. DOI: 10.1056/NEJMoa2008457. **https://www.ncbi.nlm.nih.gov/pmc/articles/PMC7200056/**

96. Munro A. The missing link? children and transmission of SARS-CoV-2. *Don't Forget the Bubbles.* 2020. **https://dontforgetthebubbles.com/the-missing-link-children-and-transmission-of-sars-cov-2/**

97. Lerer L. 'It's a pandemic, stupid.' We asked Tom Frieden, the former C.D.C. director, for some dvice. It's not all doom and gloom. *New York Times.* June 25, 2020. **https://www.nytimes.com/2020/06/25/us/politics/tom-frieden-coronavirus.html**

98. Spencer D. Masks problematic for asthmatic, autistic, deaf and hard of hearing: health advocates. *CTV News.* May 21, 2020. **https://canoe.com/news/national/masks-problematic-for-asthmatic-autistic-hearingmpaired-people**

99. COVID-19 story tip: The importance of staying cool while wearing a mask outside in the summer heat. *Johns Hopkins Medical News.* June 23, 2020. **https://www.hopkinsmedicine.org/news/newsroom/news-releases/covid-19-story-tip-the-importance-of-staying-cool-while-wearing-a-mask-outside-in-the-summer-heat**

100. Yan Y, Bayham J, Fenichel EP, Richter A. Do face masks create a false sense of security? A COVID-19 dilemma. *BioRxiv.* 2020; doi: **https://doi.org/10.1101/2020.05.23.20111302**.

101. Alvarado M. To mask or not to mask: the evolving science and policy recommendations on masks. *Local Mission.* June 9, 2020. **https://missionlocal.org/2020/06/to-mask-or-not-to-mask-the-evolving-science-and-policy-recommendations-on-masks/**

102. Chu DK, Akl EA, Duda S, et al. Physical distancing, face masks, and eye protection to prevent person-to-person transmission of SARS-CoV-2 and COVID-19: a systematic review and meta-analysis. *Lancet* 2020;395(10242):1973-1987. **https://www.thelancet.com/journals/lancet/article/PIIS01406736(20)31142-9/fulltext**

103. Gandhi M, Beyrer C, Goosby E. Masks do more than protect others during COVID-19: reducing the inoculum of SARS-CoV-2 to protect the wearer. *J Gen Intern Med.* 2020. **https://link.springer.com/article/10.1007/s11606-020-06067-8#citeas**

104. *Coronavirus disease 2019 (COVID-19) Situation Report – 66.* Geneva: WHO. March 26, 2020. **https://www.who.int/docs/default-source/coronaviruse/situation-reports/20200326-sitrep-66-covid-19.pdf?sfvrsn=9e5b8b48_2**

105. Qureshi Z, Jones N, Temple R, Larwood JPJ, Greenhalgh T, Bourouiba L. *What is the evidence to support the 2-metre social distancing rule to reduce COVID-19 transmission?* The Centre for Evidence-Based Medicine, June 22, 2020. **https://www.cebm.net/covid-19/what-is-the-evidence-to-support-the-2-metre-social-distancing-rule-to-reduce-covid-19-transmission/**

106. Netburn D. Isolation is hazardous to your health. The term 'social distancing' doesn't help. *LA Times*. March 28, 2020. **https://www.latimes.com/science/story/2020-03-28/isolation-is-hazardous-to-your-health-the-term-social-distancing-doesnt-help**

107. Allen H, Ling B, Burton W. Stop using the term 'social distancing' – start talking about 'physical distancing, social connection'. *Health Affairs blog*, April 27, 2020. **https://www.healthaffairs.org/do/10.1377/hblog20200424.213070/full/**

108. Atran S. In gods we trust. The problem of social distancing. The innate desire to help others despite the cost is one of humankind's gifts. *Psychology Today*. March 20, 2020. **https://www.psychologytoday.com/us/blog/in-gods-we-trust/202003/the-problem-social-distancing**

109. Stockman LJ, Massoudi MS, Helfand R, et al. Severe acute respiratory syndrome in children. *Pediatr Infect Dis J*. 2007;26(1):68–74. **https://pubmed.ncbi.nlm.nih.gov/17195709/**

110. Wu KJ. The coronavirus spares most kids. These theories may help explain why. *National Geographic*. March 25, 2020. **https://www.nationalgeographic.com/science/2020/03/coronavirus-spares-most-kids-these-theories-may-help-explain-why/**

111. Barber G. What's the strange ailment affecting children with Covid-19? *Wired*. May 15, 2020. **https://www.wired.com/story/whats-the-strange-ailment-affecting-kids-with-covid-19/**

112. Linas BP. I'm an epidemiologist and a dad. Here's why I think schools should reopen. Six questions about the safety of kids, teachers, and families, answered. *Vox*. July 9, 2020. **https://www.vox.com/2020/7/9/21318560/covid-19-coronavirus-us-testing-children-schools-reopening-questions**

113. Halperin DT. The case for reopening schools this fall. *Washington Post*, May 29, 2020. **https://www.washingtonpost.com/opinions/2020/05/29/case-reopening-schools-this-fall/**

114. Götzinger F, Santiago-García B, Noguera-Julián A. COVID-19 in children and adolescents in Europe: a multinational, multicentre cohort study. *Lancet Child Adol Health*. 2020. **www.thelancet.com/journals/lanchi/article/PIIS2352-4642(20)30177-2/fulltext**

115. Klausner J, Bhatia R. The way to save our kids is to reopen our schools and camps. Children are much less likely to be infected, less likely to become severely ill, and less likely to spread infection. We should let our children return to their normal lives. *Daily Beast*. May 27, 2020. **https://www.thedailybeast.com/the-way-to-save-our-kids-is-to-reopen-our-schools-and-camps**

116. Cunningham RM, Walton MA, Carter PM. The major causes of death in children and adolescents in the United States. *N Engl J Med*. 2018;379(25):2468–2475. **https://www.nejm.org/doi/full/10.1056/nejmsr1804754**

117. Pandemic update: on matters of life and death. *Private Eye*. No. 1524, July 2, 2020, p. 6. **https://www.private-eye.co.uk/issue-1524**

118. Zweig D. The case for reopening schools. *Wired*. May 11, 2020. **https://www.wired.com/story/the-case-for-reopening-schools/**

119. National Collaborating Centre for Methods and Tools. Rapid Evidence Review: What is the Specific Role of Daycares and Schools in COVID-19 Transmission? July 24, 2020. **https://www.nccmt.ca/knowledge-repositories/covid-19-rapid-evidence-service**

120. Oster E. Opening schools might be safer than you think. To gather more data, we should use

summer camps as a test. *Washington Post.* May 11, 2020.
https://webcache.googleusercontent.com/search?q=cache:-hQITPofsolJ:
https://www.washingtonpost.com/outlook/schools-open-coronavirussummer-camps-
child-care/2020/05/10/94676384-907c-11ea-a0bc-4e9ad4866d21_story.html+&c-d=1&
hl=en&ct=clnk&gl=us&client=safari

121. Coronavirus disease 2019 in children – United States, February 12-April 2, 2020.
MMWR Morb Mortal Wkly Rep 2020;69:422-426. DOI:
https://www.cdc.gov/mmwr/volumes/69/wr/mm6914e1.htm

122. Patel AB, Verma A. Nasal ACE2 levels and Covid-19 in children. *JAMA.* 2020;323(23):2386-
2387. **https://jamanetwork.com/journals/jama/fullarticle/2766522**

123. Cha AE. Forty percent of people with coronavirus infections have no symptoms. Might they be
the key to ending the pandemic? New research suggests that some of us may be partially protected
due to past encounters with common cold coronaviruses. *Washington Post.* August 8, 2020.
https://www.washingtonpost.com/health/2020/08/08/asymptomatic-coronavirus-
covid/

124. Park YJ, Choe YJ, Park O, et al. Contact tracing during coronavirus disease outbreak, South
Korea, 2020. *Emerg Infect Dis.* 2020. **https://doi.org/10.3201/eid2610.201315.**
https://wwwnc.cdc.gov/eid/article/26/10/20-1315-t1

125. Mandavilli A. Older children and the coronavirus: a new wrinkle in the debate. A new report
from South Korea throws into question an earlier finding regarding transmission by older
children. *New York Times.* August 14, 2020. **https://www.nytimes.com/2020/08/14/**
health/older-children-and-the-coronavirus-a-new-wrinkle-in-the-debate.
html?action=click&module=Well&pgtype=Homepage&section=Health

126. Achenbach J, Meckler L. Children are only half as likely to get infected with the coronavirus,
study finds. *Washington Post.* June 16, 2020. **https://www.washingtonpost.com/health/**
children-are-only-half-as-likely-to-get-infected-by-the-coronavirus-research-
shows/2020/06/16/be86aff4-afb6-11ea-856d-5054296735e5_story.html

127. Boyd C. Leading Cambridge University expert says risk for children catching COVID-19 is
'unbelievably low' and teachers are not at greater danger amid row over plans to reopen schools.
Daily Mail. May 20, 2020.
https://www.dailymail.co.uk/news/article-8340341/Leading-Cambridge-University-
expert-says-risk-children-catching-COVID-19-unbelievably-low.html

128. Coronavirus in children: risk factors, contagiousness, viral load – what we know so far as
schools consider reopening. *Reuters.* May 21, 2020. **https://www.scmp.com/lifestyle/health-**
wellness/article/3085281/coronavirus-children-risk-factors-contagiousness-viral

129. Gudbjartsson DF, Helgason, Jonsson H, et al. Spread of SARSCoV-2 in the Icelandic population. *N
Engl J Med.* 2020; 382:2302-2315. **https://www.nejm.org/doi/full/10.1056/NEJMoa2006100**

130. Zhu Y, Bloxham CJ, Hulme KD, et al. Children are unlikely to have been the primary source of
household SARS-CoV-2 infections. *MedRxiv.* doi:
https://doi.org/10.1101/2020.03.26.20044826

131. Khazan O. The school reopeners think America is forgetting about kids. Some public-health
experts say the costs of keeping schools closed outweigh the hazards of reopening them. *Atlantic.*
June 25, 2020. **https://www.theatlantic.com/health/archive/2020/06/will-schools-**
reopen-fall/613468/

132. Davidson Sorkin A. The complex question of reopening schools. *The New Yorker*. June 1, 2020. **https://www.newyorker.com/magazine/2020/06/01/the-complex-question-of-reopening-schools**

133. Reopening schools in Denmark did not worsen outbreak, data shows. *Reuters*. May 28, 2020. **https://www.reuters.com/article/us-health-coronavirus-denmark-reopening/reopening-schools-in-denmark-did-not-worsen-outbreak-data-shows-idUSKBN2341N7**

134. Crawfurd C, Hares S, Sandefur J, Minardi AL. *Back to school? Tracking COVID Cases as Schools Reopen*. Center for Global Development. May 29, 2020. **https://www.cgdev.org/blog/back-school-tracking-covid-cases-schools-reopen**

135. Pancevski B. Is it safe to reopen schools? These countries say yes. Officials say return to classrooms hasn't increased rate of coronavirus infections. *Wall St. J.* May 31, 2020. **https://www.wsj.com/articles/is-it-safe-to-reopen-schools-these-countries-say-yes-11590928949**

136. Birnbaum M. Reopened schools in Europe and Asia have largely avoided coronavirus outbreaks. They have lessons for the U.S. *New York Times*. July 11, 2020. **https://www.washingtonpost.com/world/europe/schools-reopening-coronavirus/2020/07/10/865fb3e6-c122-11ea-8908-68a2b9eae9e0_story.html**

137. *COVID-19 in Schools – The Experience in NSW. April 2020 Report 1 COVID-19 in schools – the experience in NSW*. The National Centre for Immunisation Research and Surveillance (NCIRS). April 26, 2020. **http://ncirs.org.au/sites/default/files/2020-04/NCIRS_NSW_Schools_COVID_Summary_FINAL_public_26_April_2020.pdf**

138. Fontanet A, Grant R, Tondeur L, et al. SARS-COV-2 infection in primary schools in northern France: a retrospective cohort study in an area of high transmission. Unpublished research paper, 2020. **https://www.pasteur.fr/fr/file/35404/download**

139. Reuters. German study finds low Covid-19 infection rate in schools. Tests of pupils and teachers in Saxony suggest children may act as brake on infection. Guardian. July 13, 2020. **https://www.theguardian.com/world/2020/jul/13/german-study-covid-19-infection-rate-schools-saxony**

140. Kamenetz A. What parents can learn from childcare centers that stayed open during lockdowns. *NPR*. June 24, 2020. **https://www.npr.org/2020/06/24/882316641/what-parents-can-learn-from-child-carecenters-that-stayed-open-during-lockdowns**

141. Haspel E. Childcares look safe – it's time to act like it. *Early Learning Nation*. June 10, 2020. **http://earlylearningnation.com/2020/06/opinion-child-cares-look-safe-its-time-to-act-like-it/**

142. Redlener I, Redlener KB. Today's children are the pandemic generation. *Washington Post*. May 12, 2020. **https://www.washingtonpost.com/opinions/2020/05/12/todays-children-are-pandemic-generation-millions-future-is-now-grim/**

143. Goldberg M. Remote school is a nightmare. Few in power care. Government should treat the need to reopen schools as an emergency. *New York Times*. June 29, 2020. **https://www.nytimes.com/2020/06/29/opinion/coronavirus-school-reopening.html**

144. Bauer L. The COVID-19 crisis has already left too many children hungry in America. *Brookings*. May 6, 2020. **https://www.brookings.edu/blog/up-front/2020/05/06/the-covid-19-crisis-has-already-left-too-many-children-hungry-in-america/**

145.   Lockdowns could have long-term effects on children's health. Sitting at home playing video games and eating crisps is not good for them. *Economist*. July 19, 2020. **https://www. economist.com/international/2020/07/19/lockdowns-could-have-long-term-effects-on-childrens-health**

146.   Baron EJ, Goldstein EG, Wallace C. Suffering in silence: how COVID-19 school closures inhibit the reporting of child maltreatment. *SSRN*. May 17, 2020. **https://papers.ssrn.com/sol3/ papers.cfm?abstract_id=3601399**

147.   Goldstein D. Research shows students falling months behind during virus disruptions. The abrupt switch to remote learning wiped out academic gains for many students in America, and widened racial and economic gaps. Catching up in the fall won't be easy. *New York Times*. June 5, 2020. **https://www.nytimes.com/2020/06/05/us/coronavirus-education-lost-learning.html**

148.   Dorn E, Hancock B, Sarakatsannis J, Viruleg E. COVID-19 and student learning in the United States: The hurt could last a lifetime. *McKinsey*. June 1, 2020. **https://www.mckinsey.com/ industries/public-sector/our-insights/covid-19-and-student-learning-in-the-united-states-the-hurt-could-last-a-lifetime#**

149.   Almaliti F. Life with an autistic child can be difficult. During a pandemic it can be grueling. STAT News. May 15, 2020. **https://www.statnews.com/2020/05/15/life-for-individuals-with-autism-completely-upended-by-covid-19/**

150.   Cunningham M. Swiss hugging experiment key to answers on COVID-19 risk in kids. *Sydney Morning Herald*. May 1, 2020. **https://www.smh.com.au/national/australian-experts-look-to-swissfor-answers-on-covid-19-risk-in-kids-20200501-p54oyc.html**

151.   Zhang JJ, Dong X, Cao YY, et al. Clinical characteristics of 140 patients infected with SARS-CoV-2 in Wuhan, China. *Allergy*. 2020. Feb. 19 [Online ahead of print]. **https://onlinelibrary.wiley.com/doi/full/10.1111/all.14238**

152.   Hakim D. Asthma is absent among top Covid-19 risk factors, early data shows. *New York Times*. April 16, 2020. **https://www.nytimes.com/2020/04/16/health/coronavirus-asthma-risk.html**

153.   Halpin DM, Faner R, Sibila O, Badia JR, Agusti A. Do chronic respiratory diseases or their treatment affect the risk of SARS-CoV-2 infection? *Lancet Respiratory*. 2020; **https://www.ncbi.nlm.nih.gov/pmc/articles/PMC7270536/.**

154.   Howard B. COVID-19 risks to people with asthma much lower than expected. Doctors say the lung condition isn't a major factor in serious infections. AARP. May 7, 2020. **https://www.aarp. org/health/conditions-treatments/info-2020/coronavirus-and-asthma.html**

155.   Gervasoni C, Meraviglia P, Riva A, et al. Clinical features and outcomes of HIV patients with coronavirus disease 2019. *Clinical Infectious Diseases*. 2020; **https://doi.org/10.1093/cid/ciaa579.**

156.   Nordling L, Kaiser J, Grimm D, O'Grady C, O'Grady C, Clery D. HIV and TB increase death risk from COVID-19, study finds – but not by much. *Science*. 2020, June 15, 2020. **https://www. sciencemag.org/news/2020/06/hiv-and-tb-increase-death-risk-covid-19-study-finds-not-much**

157.   Frieden T. Amateur epidemiology is deterring our covid-19 response. *Washington Post*. June 10, 2020.**https://www.washingtonpost.com/opinions/2020/06/10/how-amateur-epidemiology-can-hurt-our-covid-19-response/**

158. Coronavirus (COVID-19) death rate in countries with confirmed deaths and over 1,000 reported cases as of June 26, 2020, by country. *Statista*. 2020; **https://www.statista.com/statistics/1105914/coronavirus-death-rates-worldwide/**

159. Regalado A. Blood tests show 14% of people are now immune to covid-19 in one town in Germany. *MIT Technology Review*. April 9, 2020. **https://www.technologyreview.com/2020/04/09/999015/blood-tests-show-15-of-people-are-now-immune-to-covid-19-in-one-town-in-germany/**

160. *Number of coronavirus cases by age group* (for various countries). Statista. May 16, 2020. **https://www.statista.com/statistics/1107905/number-of-coronavirus-cases-in-sweden-by-age-groups/**

161. Quinton S. Staffing nursing homes was hard before the pandemic. Now it's even tougher. *Fierce Healthcare*. May 18, 2020. **https://www.pewtrusts.org/en/research-and-analysis/blogs/stateline/2020/05/18/staffing-nursing-homes-was-hard-before-the-pandemic-now-its-even-tougher**

162. Woodward A, Secon H. Fauci said he's 'willing to bet anything' that people who recover from the new coronavirus are 'really protected from reinfection'. *Business Insider*. March 28, 2020. **https://www.businessinsider.com/coronavirus-fauci-those-who-recover-will-be-immune-2020-3**

163. Sample I. Immunity to Covid-19 could be lost in months, UK study suggests. *Guardian*. July 12, 2020. **https://www.theguardian.com/world/2020/jul/12/immunity-to-covid-19-could-be-lost-in-months-uk-study-suggests**

164. Mandavilli A. This trawler's haul: evidence that antibodies block the coronavirus. Three crew members aboard were spared when the virus spread through the boat. They were the only ones who had antibodies at the beginning of the trip. *New York Times*. August 19, 2020. **https://www.nytimes.com/2020/08/19/health/coronavirus-fishing-boat.html**

165. Yong E. Immunology is where intuition goes to die. Which is too bad because we really need to understand how the immune system reacts to the coronavirus. *The Atlantic*, August 5, 2020. **https://www.theatlantic.com/health/archive/2020/08/covid-19-immunity-is-the-pandemics-central-mystery/614956/**

166. Draulans D. 'Finally, a virus got me.' Scientist who fought Ebola and HIV reflects on facing death from COVID-19. *Science*. May 8, 2020. **https://www.sciencemag.org/news/2020/05/finally-virus-got-me-scientist-who-fought-ebola-and-hiv-reflects-facing-death-covid-19**

167. Parshley L. The emerging long-term complications of Covid-19, explained. "It is a true roller coaster of symptoms and severities, with each new day offering many unknowns." *Vox*. June 12, 2020. **https://www.vox.com/2020/5/8/21251899/coronavirus-long-term-effects-symptoms**

168. Belluck P. Here's what recovery from Covid-19 looks like for many survivors. Continuing shortness of breath, muscle weakness, flashbacks, mental fogginess and other symptoms may plague patients for a long time. *New York Times*. July 1, 2020. **https://www.nytimes.com/2020/07/01/health/coronavirus-recovery-survivors.html**

169. Economist. When covid-19 becomes a chronic illness. Scientists are investigating why some people suffer with the virus for many months. *Economist*. August 22, 2020. **https://www.economist.com/science-and-technology/2020/08/22/when-covid-19-becomes-a-chronic-illness**

170. Geddes, L. Why strange and debilitating coronavirus symptoms can last for months. *New Scientist*. June 24, 2020. **https://www.newscientist.com/article/mg24632881-400-why-strange-and-debilitatingcoronavirus-symptoms-can-last-for-months/**

171. Sellers SA, Hagan R, Hayden F, Fischer WA II. The hidden burden of influenza: A review of the extra-pulmonary complications of influenza infection. *Influenza Other Resp Viruses*. 2017;11:372-393. **https://doi.org/10.1111/irv.12470**.

172. Holloway H. Quarantine row. Scientists say 14-day quarantine rule to fight coronavirus spread 'makes no sense' as calls grow for it to be scrapped. *The Sun*. June 4, 2020. **https://www.thesun.co.uk/news/11779198/14-day-quarantine-coronavirus-makes-no-sense/**

173. Elegant N. How the world agreed on a 14-day coronavirus quarantine and how to shorten it. *Forbes*. June 8, 2020. **https://fortune.com/2020/06/08/14-days-coronavirus-2-week-quarantine-questions-covid-19/**

174. Auwaerter PG. Coronavirus COVID-19 (SARS-CoV-2). *Johns Hopkins ABX Guide*. June 28, 2020. **https://www.hopkinsguides.com/hopkins/view/Johns_Hopkins_ABX_Guide/540747/all/Corona-virus_COVID_19__SARS_CoV_2_?q=covid+period+quarantine**

175. Osterholm MT, Olshaker M. Facing covid-19 reality: a national lockdown is no cure. *Washington Post*. March 21, 2020. **https://webcache.googleusercontent.com/search?q=cache:W8bKORafDV-4J:https://www.washingtonpost.com/opinions/2020/03/21/facing-covid-19-reality-national-lock-down-is-no-cure/+&cd=1&hl=en&ct=clnk&gl=us&client=safari**

176. Katz D. Is our fight against coronavirus worse than the disease? *New York Times*. March 20, 2020. **https://www.nytimes.com/2020/03/20/opinion/coronavirus-pandemic-social-distancing.html**

177. Ioannidis JP. A fiasco in the making? As the coronavirus pandemic takes hold, we are making decisions without reliable data. *STATNews*. March 17, 2020. **https://www.statnews.com/ 2020/03/17/a-fiasco-in-the-making-as-the-coronavirus-pandemic-takes-hold-we-are-making-decisions-without-reliable-data/**

178. Hotez P. COVID-19 vaccine in 12-18 months would be 'unprecedented'. **https://www.youtube.com/watch?v=VI-xhMYhvLs**

179. Goldstein J. 68% have antibodies in this clinic. Can neighborhood beat a next wave? Data from those tested at a storefront medical office in Queens is leading to a deeper understanding of the outbreak's scope in New York. *New York Times*. July 9, 2020. **https://www.nytimes.com/2020/07/09/nyregion/nyc-coronavirus-antibodies.html?referringSource=articleShare**

180. Mandavilli Covid-19: What if 'herd immunity' is closer than scientists thought? In what may be the world's most important math puzzle, researchers are trying to figure out how many people in a community must be immune before the coronavirus fades. *The New York Times*. August 17, 2020. **https://www.nytimes.com/2020/08/17/health/coronavirus-herd-immunity.html**

181. Hamblin J. A new understanding of herd immunity. The portion of the population that needs to get sick is not fixed. We can change it. *Atlantic*. July 13, 2020. **https://www.theatlantic.com/health/archive/2020/07/herd-immunity-coronavirus/614035/**

182. Mandavilli A, Thomas K. Will an antibody test allow us to go back to school or work? *New York Times*. April 10, 2020. **https://www.nytimes.com/2020/04/10/health/coronavirus-antibody-test.html**

183. Kottasová I. Welcome to the whack-a-mole stage of coronavirus. *CNN*. June 24, 2020. **http:// www.cnn.com/2020/06/24/europe/coronavirus-germany-outbreaks-intl-grm/index. html**

184. Hodgins S, Saad A. Will the higher-income country blueprint for COVID-19 work in low and lower middle-income countries? *Glob Health Sci Pract*. 2020;8(2):136-143. **https://doi. org/10.9745/GHSP-D-20-00217**

185. Mehtar S, PreiserW, Lakhe NA, et al. Limiting the spread of COVID-19 in Africa: one size mitigation strategies do not fit all countries. *Lancet Glob Health*. April 28, 2020. **https://www. ncbi.nlm.nih.gov/pmc/articles/PMC7195296/**

186. Cash R, Patel V. Has COVID-19 subverted global health? *Lancet*. May 5, 2020. **https://www. ncbi.nlm.nih.gov/pmc/articles/PMC7200122/**

187. Loayza, Norman V. *Costs and Trade-Offs in the Fight Against the COVID-19 Pandemic: A Developing Country Perspective (English)*. Research & Policy Briefs; no. 35. 2020. World Bank Group, Washington, D.C. **http://documents.worldbank.org/curated/ en/799701589552654684/Costs-and-Trade-Offs-in-the-Fight-Against-the-COVID-19- Pandemic-A-Developing-Country-Perspective**

188. Barasa E, Mothupi MC, Guleid F, et al. *DFID Policy Brief Rapid Review of Physical Distancing in Africa*. FfID, London. May 15, 2020. **https://reliefweb.int/report/world/rapid-review- physical-distancing-and-alternative-disease-control-measures-south-asia-15**

189. Walker D, Chi YL, Poli F, Chalkidou K. *A Tool to Estimate the Net Health Impact of COVID-19 Policies*. Center for Global Development, Washington DC. May 26, 2020. **https://www.cgdev. org/blog/tool-estimate-net-health-impact-covid-19-policies**

190. Heath A. Sweden's success shows the true cost of our arrogant, failed establishment. Shocking incompetence has unnecessarily wiped billions of pounds from the UK economy. *Telegraph*. August 12, 2020. **https://www.telegraph.co.uk/news/2020/08/12/swedens-success- shows-true-cost-arrogant-failed-establishment/**

191. Leatherby L, McCann A. Sweden stayed open. A deadly month shows the risks. Sweden's outbreak has been far deadlier than those of its neighbors, but it's still better off than many countries that enforced strict lockdowns. *New York Times*. May 15, 2020. **https://www.nytimes. com/interactive/2020/05/15/world/europe/sweden-coronavirus-deaths.html**

192. Tran AB, Shapiro L, Brown E. Pandemic's overall death toll in U.S. likely surpassed 100,000 weeks ago. A state-by-state analysis shows that deaths officially attributed to Covid-19 only partially account for unusually high mortality during the pandemic. *Washington Post*. May 30, 2020. **https://www. washingtonpost.com/graphics/2020/investigations/coronavirus-excess-deaths-may/**

193. Ritchie H, Roser M, Ortiz-Ospina E, Hasell J. Excess mortality from the Coronavirus pandemic (COVID-19). *Our World in Data*. **https://ourworldindata.org/excess-mortality-covid**

194. Tracking covid-19 excess deaths across countries; official covid-19 death tolls still under-count the true number of fatalities. *Economist*. April 16, 2020. **https://www.economist.com/graphic- detail/2020/04/16/tracking-covid-19-excess-deaths-across-countries**

195. Many covid deaths in care homes are unrecorded. *Economist*. May 9, 2020. **https://www. economist.com/europe/2020/05/09/many-covid-deaths-in-care-homes-are-unrecorded**

196. Potter B. Two-thirds of region's COVID-19 deaths have occurred in long-term care facilities.

Inside NOVA. Jun 19, 2020 **https://www.insidenova.com/headlines/two-thirds-of-regions-covid-19-deaths-have-occurred-in-long-term-care-facilities/article_630bf5f6-b260-11ea-9f4d-4b58e8891e9e.html**

197. Rothschild R. The hidden flaw in Sweden's anti-lockdown strategy. The government expects citizens to freely follow its advice—but not all ethnic groups have equal access to expertise. *Foreign Policy*. April 21, 2020. **https://foreignpolicy.com/2020/04/21/sweden-coronavirus-anti-lockdown-immigrants/**

198. McCarthy M. COVID-19: How far away are we from herd immunity? *Statista*. May 29, 2020. **https://www.statista.com/chart/21866/estimated-share-of-the-population-with-covid-19-antibodies/**

199. Greenfield D. Sweden cared more about Islamophobia than saving elderly in nursing homes from Coronavirus. *FrontPage Mag*. May 12, 2020. **https://www.frontpagemag.com/fpm/2020/05/sweden-cared-more-about-islamophobia-saving-daniel-greenfield/**

200. Keyton D. Coronavirus takes a toll in Sweden's immigrant community. *AP News*. May 9, 2020. **https://apnews.com/1d7916cf6e48b7a231b894ef9cda1a19**

201. Gjevori E. Can Sweden do more to protect the Somali community? *TRT World*. June 12, 2020. **https://www.trtworld.com/magazine/coronavirus-can-sweden-do-more-to-protect-the-somali-community-37227**

202. Anthony Mounts. Personal communication, July 6, 2020. WHO data indicating that between 2%-26% of Somalis received the tuberculosis (BCG) vaccine during the 1980s, compared with 30%-72% of Kenyans and 10%-72% of Ghanaians during the same period. Levels fluctuated greatly from year to year, but the Somalis overall had far lower coverage during all years. Unusually high Covid-19 deaths among Somalis have been reported elsewhere, including Finland and Norway: Keyton D. Coronavirus takes a toll in Sweden's immigrant community. *Associated Press*. May 9, 2020. **https://abcnews.go.com/International/wireStory/coronavirus-takes-toll-swedens-immigrant-community-70593594**

203. Mascarenhas L. More evidence emerges that a TB vaccine might help fight coronavirus. *CNN*. July 10, 2020. **https://edition.cnn.com/2020/07/10/health/tb-bcg-vaccine-coronavirus-study/index.html**

204. Chumakov K, Benn CS, Aaby P, Kottilil S, Gallo R. Can existing live vaccines prevent COVID-19? *Science*. 2020;368(6496):1187-1188. **https://science.sciencemag.org/content/368/6496/1187**

205. Moyer MW. Could 'innate immunology' save us from the coronavirus? Researchers are testing whether decades-old vaccines for polio and tuberculosis could protect against infection. *New York Times*. May 1, 2020. **https://www.nytimes.com/2020/05/01/opinion/sunday/coronavirus-vaccine-innate-immunity.html?action=click&module=RelatedLinks&pgtype=Article**

206. Wingfield-Hayes R. Coronavirus: Japan's mysteriously low virus death rate. *BBC News*, July 4, 2020. **https://www.bbc.com/news/world-asia-53188847**

207. Halperin DT. The Covid-19 lockdown "natural experiment" that has already been conducted. *SocArXiv*. doi:10.31235/osf.io/jzhe2. **https://osf.io/preprints/socarxiv/jzhe2/**

208. Rodgers TJ. Do lockdowns save many lives? In most places, the data say no. *Wall Street Journal*. April 26, 2020. **https://www.wsj.com/articles/do-lockdowns-save-many-lives-is-most-places-the-data-say-no-11587930911**

209.   Kupferschmidt K. Why do some COVID-19 patients infect many others, whereas most don't spread the virus at all? *Science*. May. 19, 2020. **https://www.sciencemag.org/news/2020/05/why-do-some-covid-19-patients-infect-many-others-whereas-most-don-t-spread-virus-all**

210.   Li W, Zhang B, Lu J, et al. The characteristics of household transmission of COVID-19. *Clin Infect Dis*. April 17, 2020. **https://academic.oup.com/cid/article/doi/10.1093/cid/ciaa450/5821281**

211.   Qian H, Miao T, Liu L, Zheng X, Luo D, Li Y. Indoor transmission of SARS-CoV-2. *medRxiv*. 2020; **https://doi.org/10.1101/2020.04.04.20053058.**

212.   Nishiura H, Oshitani H, Kobayashi T, et al. Closed environments facilitate secondary transmission of coronavirus disease 2019 (COVID-19). MedRxiv. 2020. doi: **https://doi.org/10.1101/2020.02.28.20029272 https://www.medrxiv.org/content/10.1101/2020.02.28.20029272v2**

213.   Allen JG, Macomber JD. Healthy Buildings: *How Indoor Spaces Drive Performance and Productivity*. 2020. **https://www.amazon.com/dp/0674237978/ref=cm_sw_r_other_apa_i_JOTyFb6XQORQB**

214.   Hilgers L. How two waves of coronavirus cases swept through the Texas panhandle. *New Yorker*. July 10, 2020. **https://www.newyorker.com/magazine/dispatch/how-two-waves-of-coronavirus-cases-swept-through-the-texas-panhandle**

215.   Perez M. 87% of meatpacking workers infected with coronavirus have been racial and ethnic minorities, CDC says. *Forbes*. July 7, 2020. **https://www.forbes.com/sites/mattperez/2020/07/07/87-of-meatpacking-workers-infected-with-coronavirus-have-been-racial-and-ethnic-minorities-cdc-says/#cb06883634f5**

216.   Molten M. Why meatpacking plants have become Covid-19 hot spots. Wired. May 7, 2020. **https://www.wired.com/story/why-meatpacking-plants-have-become-covid-19-hot-spots/**

217.   Williams T, Seline L, Griesbach R. Coronavirus cases rise sharply in prisons even as they plateau nationwide. *New York Times*. June 16, 2020. **https://www.nytimes.com/2020/06/16/us/coronavirus-inmates-prisons-jails.html**

218.   San Quentin: Covid-19 cases at California prison surge to 1,000. *Guardian*. June 29, 2020. **https://www.theguardian.com/us-news/2020/jun/29/san-quentin-coronavirus-cases-covid-19**

219.   Sternlicht A. Prisoners 550% more likely to get Covid-19, 300% more likely to die, new study shows. *Forbes*. July 8, 2020. **https://www.forbes.com/sites/alexandrasternlicht/2020/07/08/prisoners-550-more-likely-to-get-covid-19-300-more-likely-to-die-new-study-shows/#4a43f7d63a72**

220.   Lewis A. What we do and don't know about the links between air pollution and coronavirus. *The Conversation*. **https://theconversation.com/what-we-do-and-dont-know-about-the-linksbetween-airpollution-and-coronavirus-137746**

221. Yglesias M. The successful Asian coronavirus-fighting strategy America refuses to embrace. Other countries have had better results putting sick people into isolation instead of sending them home to potentially infect their family. *Vox.* April 28, 2020. **https://www.vox.com/2020/4/28/21238456/centralized-isolation-coronavirus-hong-kong-korea**

222. Kolbert E. How Iceland beat the coronavirus. The country didn't just manage to flatten the curve; it virtually eliminated it. *New Yorker.* June 1, 2020. **https://www.newyorker.com/magazine/2020/06/08/how-iceland-beat-the-coronavirus**

223. *Iceland Eases Restrictions All Children's Activities Back to Normal.* Iceland Ministry for Foreign Affairs, Ministry of Justice, Ministry of Health. May 06, 2020. **https://www.government.is/news/article/2020/05/06/Iceland-eases-restrictions-all-childrens-activities-back-to-normal/**

224. Yudistira N, Sumitro SB, Nahas A, Riama NF. UV light influences covid-19 activity through big data: trade-offs between northern subtropical, tropical, and southern subtropical countries. *medRxiv.* 2020. **https://www.medrxiv.org/content/10.1101/2020.04.30.20086983v3**

225. Bukhari Q, Jameel Y. Will coronavirus pandemic diminish by summer? *Massachusetts Institute of Technology.* March 17, 2020. **https://climaya.com/wp-content/uploads/2020/03/SSRN-id3558757.pdf**

226. Wu Y, Jing W, Liu J, et al. Effects of temperature and humidity on the daily new cases and new deaths of COVID-19 in 166 countries. *Sci Total Environ.* 2020;729:139051. **https://www.sciencedirect.com/science/article/pii/S0048969720325687**

227. Loria K. Being outside can improve memory, fight depression, and lower blood pressure — here are 12 science-backed reasons to spend more time outdoors. *Business Insider.* April 22, 2020. **https://www.businessinsider.com/why-spending-more-time-outside-is-healthy-2017-7**

228. Popkin G. Don't cancel the outdoors; we need it to stay sane. *Washington Post.* March 20, 2020. **https://www.washingtonpost.com/outlook/2020/03/24/dontcancel-outdoors-we-need-them-stay-sane/**

229. Kolata G. In Norway, gymgoers avoid infections as virus recedes. In an unusual experiment, researchers found no coronavirus infections among thousands of people allowed to return to their gyms. *New York Times.* June 25, 2020. **https://www.nytimes.com/2020/06/25/health/coronavirus-gyms-fitness.html**

230. Gathara P. Kenya is turning a public health crisis into a law-and-order one. *Washington Post.* May 7, 2020. **https://www.washingtonpost.com/opinions/2020/05/07/kenya-is-turning-public-health-crisis-into-law-and-order-one/**

231. Kenya: Police brutality in the battle against coronavirus in Mathare. *BBC News.* June 15, 2020. **https://www.bbc.co.uk/news/world-africa-53025934**

232. Jones S. Gov. Cuomo on ventilator situation: 'We're ok, and we have some in reserve'. *CNS News.* April 7, 2020. **https://www.cnsnews.com/article/national/susan-jones/gov-cuomo-ventilator-situation-were-ok-and-we-have-some-reserve**

233. Sklar J. Why rural hospitals may not survive COVID-19. With fear of COVID-19 keeping many routine visitors away, rural hospitals have too few patients to stay afloat financially, and virtual medicine isn't saving them. *National Geographic.* June 2, 2020. **https://www.nationalgeographic.com/science/2020/06/why-rural-hospitals-may-not-survive-coronavirus-telemedicine/**

234. Bhatia R. Public Epidemiology: Untangling COVID-19 (blog). **https://publicepi.org/**

235. McNeil D. A simple way to save lives as Covid-19 hits poorer nations. Aid agencies are scrambling to get oxygen equipment to low-income countries where the coronavirus is rapidly spreading. *New York Times.* June 23, 2020. **https://www.nytimes.com/2020/06/23/health/coronavirus-oxygen-africa.html**

236. de Freytas-Tamura K, Hubler S, Fuchs S, Montgomery D. Like 'a bus accident a day': hospitals strain under new flood of Covid-19 patients. I.C.U. units are reaching capacity. Nurses are falling sick, contributing to shortages. The new coronavirus spikes are challenging hospitals across the United States. *New York Times.* July 9, 2020. **https://www.nytimes.com/2020/07/09/us/coronavirus-hospitals-capacity.html?action=click&module=Top%20Stories&pgtype=Homepage**

237. *Overview of TMC ICU Bed Capacity and Occupancy.* Houston: Texas Medical Center. 2020. **https://www.tmc.edu/coronavirus-updates/overview-of-tmc-icu-bed-capacity-and-occupancy/**

238. Goodman CK. In Florida hospitals, lessons learned from more than 3,300 deaths. *South Florida Sun Sentinel.* June 27, 2020. **https://www.sun-sentinel.com/coronavirus/fl-ne-coronavirus-florida-hospitalization-20200627-jnttxqim7zgwdicgxygfsstysq-story.html**

239. A younger and less sick wave of COVID patients is surging through Miami-Dade hospitals. *Miami Herald.* June 23, 2020. **https://www.miamiherald.com/search/?q=covid+hospital+stays#storylink=cpy**

240. Pancevski B. Forgotten pandemic offers contrast to today's coronavirus lockdowns. *Wall Street Journal.* April 24, 2020. **https://www.wsj.com/articles/forgotten-pandemic-offers-contrast-to-todays-coronavirus-lockdowns-11587720625**

241. United Nations News. Chronic illnesses: UN stands up to stop 41 million avoidable deaths per year. *UN News.* September 27, 2018. **https://news.un.org/en/story/2018/09/1021132**

242. Finkelstein, EA, Trogdon JG, Cohen W, Dietz W. Annual medica spending attributable to obesity: payer-and service-specific estimates. *Health Aff.* 2009;28(5):w822–w831. **https://www.healthaffairs.org/doi/full/10.1377/hlthaff.28.5.w822#:~:text=Across%20all%20payers%2C%20our%20results,based%20on%20the%20NHEA%20data.**

243. Halperin D. Puerto Rico's man-made disasters will kill more people than natural catastrophes. *Miami Herald.* January 20, 2020. **https://www.miamiherald.com/opinion/op-ed/article239463738.html**

244. Van Beusekom M. CDC: Pregnant women with COVID-19 face more critical care. CIDRAP News. June 25, 2020. **https://www.cidrap.umn.edu/news-perspective/2020/06/cdc-pregnant-women-covid-2019-face-more-critical-care**

245. Rettner R. Pregnancy may make COVID-19 more severe, new study suggests. *Live Science.* June 25, 2020. **https://www.livescience.com/covid-19-pregnancy-severe-illness-cdc.html**

246. de Freytas-Tamura K. Pregnant and scared of 'Covid Hospitals,' they're giving birth at home. *New York Times.* April 21, 2020. **https://www.nytimes.com/2020/04/21/nyregion/coronavirus-home-births.html**

247. Texas Coronavirus map and case count; new reported deaths by day in Texas. *New York Times.* July 8, 2020. **https://www.nytimes.com/interactive/2020/us/texas-coronavirus-cases. html**

248. *Texas Health Data; Selected Causes of Death for Texas Residents.* Texas Department of State Health Services, Austin; 2020. **http://healthdata.dshs.texas.gov/dashboard/births-and-deaths/deaths-all-ages**

249. Bernstein B. More covid-19 patients are surviving ventilators in the ICU. *Washington Post.* July 3, 2020. **https://www.washingtonpost.com/health/more-covid-19-patients-are-surviving-ventilators-in-the-icu/2020/07/03/2e3c3534-bbca-11ea-8cf5-9c1b8d7f84c6_ story.html?utm_campaign=wp_evening_edition&utm_medium=email&utm_ source=newsletter&wpisrc=nl_evening**

250. Edwards E. What ICU doctors have learned about COVID-19 — and how they're prepared for a 2nd wave. From keeping patients off ventilators to trusting that their PPE will keep them safe. *NBC News.* June 13, 2020. **https://www.nbcnews.com/health/health-news/what-icu-doctors-have-learned-aboutcovid-19-how-they-n1225801**

251. Bennhold K. A German exception? Why the country's coronavirus death rate is low. The pandemic has hit Germany hard, with more than 100,000 people infected. But the percentage of fatal cases has been remarkably low compared to those in many neighboring countries. *New York Times.* April 4, 2020. **https://www.nytimes.com/2020/04/04/world/europe/germany-coronavirus-death-rate.html**

252. Napton S. Lockdown may cost 200,000 lives, government report shows; research shines a light on the reasons why the Government has been keen to lift lockdown, in spite of experts claiming it happened too soon. *Telegraph.* July 19, 2020. **https://www.telegraph.co.uk/ news/2020/07/19/lockdown-may-cost-200k-lives-government-report-shows/**

253. Jan T, Clement S. Hispanics are almost twice as likely as whites to have lost their jobs amid pandemic. *Washington Post.* May 6, 2020. **https://www.washingtonpost.com/ business/2020/05/06/layoffs-race-poll-coronavirus/**

254. Leatherby L. Coronavirus is hitting black business owners hardest. The coronavirus pandemic will shutter many small businesses. And early evidence shows it is disproportionately hurting black-owned small businesses. *New York Times.* June 18, 2020. **https://www.nytimes.com/ interactive/2020/06/18/us/coronavirus-black-owned-small-business.html**

255. Pifer R. 27 million Americans may have lost job-based health insurance due to COVID-19 downturn. *Health Care Dive.* May 13, 2020. **https://www.healthcaredive.com/news/27m-americans-may-havelost-job-based-health-insurance-due-to-covid-19-down/577852/**

256. Garfield R, Claxton G, Damico A, Levitt L. Eligibility for ACA health coverage following job loss. *Kaiser Family Foundation.* May 13, 2020. **https://www.kff.org/coronavirus-covid-19/issue-brief/eligibility-for-aca-health-coverage-following-job-loss/**

257. Cota-Robles M. U.S. sees spike in deadly crashes during COVID-19 lockdown, data shows. There's been a rise in deadly crashes in California while people have been staying home because of the novel coronavirus, according to new data. *ABC News.* May 20, 2020. **https://abc7.com/ traffic-fatalities-california-highway-patrol-speeding-covid-19/6198603/**

258. Carey, Benedict. Is the pandemic sparking suicide?" *The New York Times*, May 19, 2020. **https:// www.nytimes.com/2020/05/19/health/pandemic-coronavirus-suicide-health.html**

259. Adam D. The hellish side of handwashing: how coronavirus is affecting people with OCD. *Guardian*. March 29, 2020. **https://www.theguardian.com/society/2020/mar/13/why-regular-handwashing-canbe-bad-advice-for-patients**

260. Lawrence E. COVID-19 worsens obsessive-compulsive disorder—but therapy offers coping skills. The pandemic has heightened OCD phobias such as fear of germs. Yet some patients say experience with anxiety, and treatment for it, gives them an advantage. *Scientific Amer.* June 18, 2020. **https://www.scientificamerican.com/article/covid-19-worsens-obsessive-compulsive-disorder-but-therapy-offers-coping-skills1/**

261. Honos-Webb L. Covid-19 induced "ADHD": finding focus in a global pandemic. Massive disruptions and distractions can make you feel like you have ADHD. *Psychology Today.* April 13, 2020. **https://www.psychologytoday.com/us/blog/the-gift-adhd/202004/covid-19-induced-adhd-finding-focus-in-global-pandemic**

262. Prasai S. Covid-19 in Nepal: where are we after 9 weeks of lock-down? *New Spotlight Nepal.* May 19, 2020. **https://www.spotlightnepal.com/2020/05/19/covid-19-nepal-where-are-we-after-9-weeks-lockdown/**

263. Oestericher D. When lockdown becomes a death sentence: The Coronavirus response in the developing world. *The Politic.* May 9, 2020. **https://thepolitic.org/when-lockdown-becomes-a-death-sentence-the-coronavirus-response-in-the-developing-world/**

264. Win TL, Harrisberg K. Africa faces 'hunger pandemic' as coronavirus destroys jobs and fuels poverty. *Reuters.* April 24, 2020. **https://www.reuters.com/article/us-health-coronavirus-africa-hunger-feat/africa-faces-hunger-pandemic-as-coronavirus-destroys-jobs-and-fuels-poverty-idUSKCN22629V**

265. WHO estimates malaria deaths could double because of interruptions caused by COVID-19. *HEALIO Infectious Disease News.* April 20, 2020. **https://www.healio.com/infectious/disease/emerging-diseases/news/online/%7Bc34b63f9-b383-4a42-8162-527965c684fa%7D/**

266. Ford L. Millions predicted to develop tuberculosis as result of Covid-19 lockdown. *Guardian.* May 6, 2020. **https://www.theguardian.com/global-development/2020/may/06/millions-develop-tuberculosis-tb-covid-19-lockdown**

267. Roberts L. Polio, measles, other diseases set to surge as COVID-19 forces suspension of vaccination campaigns. Science. April 9, 2020. **https://www.sciencemag.org/news/2020/04/polio-measles-other-diseases-set-surge-covid-19-forces-suspension-vaccination-campaigns**

268. Stover J, Chagoma N, Taramusi I, Teng Y, Glaubius R, Mahiane SG. Estimation of the potential impact of COVID-19 responses on the HIV epidemic: analysis using the Goals Model. *MedRxiv.* 2020. doi: **https://doi.org/10.1101/2020.05.04.20090399**; **https://www.medrxiv.org/content/10.1101/2020.05.04.20090399v1**

269. Hogan AB, Jewell B, Sherrard-Smith E, et al. *Report 19: The Potential Impact of the COVID-19 Epidemic on HIV, TB and Malaria in Low-and Middle-Income Countries,* MRC Centre for Global Infectious Dis Anal. 2020; doi:10.25561/78670 **https://www.imperial.ac.uk/mrc-global-infectious-disease-analysis/covid-19/report-19-hiv-tb-malaria/**

270. Santoli JM, Lindley MC, DeSilva MB, et al. Effects of the COVID-19 pandemic on routine pediatric vaccine ordering and administration-United States, 2020. *MMWR Morb Mortal Wkly Rep.* 2020;69:591–593. **https://www.cdc.gov/mmwr/volumes/69/wr/mm6919e2.htm**

271. Fernandez M. Vaccinations are plummeting amid coronavirus pandemic. A decline in pediatric care during the pandemic has put a lot of children behind the curve on routine vaccinations. *Axios*. June 20, 2020. **https://www.axios.com/children-coronavirus-vaccinations-d2e86bd2-034e-4cc9-82b9-156fb9621f4f.html**

272. Roberton T, Carter ED, Chou VB. Early estimates of the indirect effects of the COVID-19 pandemic on maternal and child mortality in low-income and middle-income countries: a modelling study. *Lancet Glob Health*. 2020. **https://www.thelancet.com/journals/langlo/article/PIIS2214-109X(20)30238-2/fulltext**

273. Santoshini S. Family planning efforts upended by the coronavirus: in India and around the world, community health workers are being rerouted to deal with the pandemic—with dangerous results. *Foreign Policy*. May 13, 2020. **https://foreignpolicy.com/2020/05/13/india-family-planning-upended-coronavirus-women-sexual-reproductive-health/**

274. Miller A, Reandelar MJ, Fasciglione K, Roumenova V, Li Y, Otazu GH. Correlation between universal BCG vaccination policy and reduced morbidity and mortality for COVID-19: an epidemiological study. *medRxiv*. March 2020. doi: https://doi.org/10.1101/2020.03.24.20042937 **https://www.medrxiv.org/content/10.1101/2020.03.24.20042937v1**

275. King A. An old TB vaccine finds new life in coronavirus trials. *The Scientist*. May 4, 2020. **https://www.the-scientist.com/news-opinion/an-old-tb-vaccine-finds-new-lifein-coronavirus-trials-67504**

276. Bao L, DengW, Gao H, et al. Reinfection could not occur in SARSCoV-2 infected rhesus macaques. *bioRxiv*. 2020; doi: **https://doi.org/10.1101/2020.03.13.990226 https://www.biorxiv.org/content/10.1101/2020.03.13.990226v1**

277. Payne D. Doctors around world say COVID-19 may be losing its potency, becoming less deadly. Doctors in Italy, Israel and U.S. say the coronavirus may be losing its potency and becoming less deadly even as it spreads. *Just the News*, June 8, 2020. **https://justthenews.com/politics-policy/coronavirus/doctors-around-world-say-covid-19-losing-its-potency-becoming-less**

278. Kaplan S, Achenbach J. This coronavirus mutation has taken over the world. Scientists are trying to understand why. *Washington Post*. June 29, 2020. **https://www.washingtonpost.com/science/2020/06/29/coronavirus-mutation-science/?arc404=true**

279. Janes C. Experts dispute reports that coronavirus is becoming less lethal. *Washington Post*. June 1, 2020. **https://www.washingtonpost.com/health/experts-dispute-reports-coronavirus-is-becoming-less-lethal/2020/06/01/8f8ace7c-a432-11ea-b619-3f9133bbb482_story.html**

280. Worldometer Coronavirus Information, Deaths per Day. July 7, 2020. **https://www.worldometers.info/coronavirus/**

281. Hashim A. The curious case of South Asia's 'low' coronavirus deaths. Varying demographics and differences in disease exposure could explain lower mortality rate in South Asian countries. *Aljazeera*. May 18, 2020. **https://www.aljazeera.com/news/2020/05/curious-case-south-asia-coronavirus-deaths-200518090320358.html**

282. Altstedter A, Pandya D. Herd immunity seems to be developing in Mumbai's poorest areas. Growing herd immunity may also be behind the dip in cases in the capital city of New Delhi, chairman of the Scientific Advisory Committee of National Institute of Epidemiology said. *Bloomberg*, July 29, 2020. **https://www.ndtv.com/india-news/herd-immunity-against-coronavirus-seems-to-be-developing-in-mumbais-poorest-areas-2271006**

283. Models project sharp rise in deaths as states reopen. *New York Times.* May 4, 2020. **https://www.nytimes.com/2020/05/04/us/coronavirus-live-updates.html**

284. Steinhauer J. The nation wanted to eat out again. Everyone has paid the price. *New York Times.* August 12, 2020. **https://www.nytimes.com/2020/08/12/health/Covid-restaurants-bars.html**

285. Bosman J, Mervosh S. As virus surges, younger people account for 'disturbing' number of cases. People in their 20s, 30s and 40s account for a growing proportion of the cases in many places, raising fears that asymptomatic young people are helping to fuel the virus's spread. *New York Times,* June 25, 2020. **https://www.nytimes.com/2020/06/25/us/coronavirus-cases-young-people.html**

286. Bernstein L, Weiner R, Achenbach J. Coronavirus deaths lag behind surging infections but may catch up soon *Washington Post.* June 24, 2020. **https://www.washingtonpost.com/health/coronavirus-deaths-lag-behind-surging-infections-but-may-catch-up-soon/2020/06/24/22263b50-b620-11ea-a510-55bf26485c93_story.html?utm_campaign=wp_politics_%20am&utm_medium=email&utm_source=newsletter&wpisrc=nl_politics**

287. Wu K. U.S. coronavirus cases are rising sharply, but deaths are still down. This seemingly counterintuitive trend might not last, experts said. But the nation can still learn from the decline. *New York Times.* July 3,2020. **https://www.nytimes.com/2020/07/03/health/coronavirus-mortality-testing.html**

288. Board T. Opinion: coping with covid-19. *Wall St J.* June 24, 2020. **https://www.wsj.com/articles/coping-with-covid-19-11593041285**

289. Campbell D. Screen survivors of Covid-19 for PTSD, say mental health experts. Specialists say condition likely to be widespread among those admitted to hospital. *Guardian.* June 28, 2020. **https://www.theguardian.com/world/2020/jun/28/screen-survivors-of-covid-19-for-ptsd-say-mental-health-experts**

290. Rhoton B. PTSD from COVID: the aftershock no one talks about. WebMD. July 07, 2020. **https://blogs.webmd.com/my-experience/20200707/ptsd-from-covid-the-aftershock-no-one-talks-about?ecd=wnl_spr_070720&ctr=wnl-spr-070720_nsl-LeadModule_cta&mb=OwCxcQ2sCvvWcxMEQZbE-F3g0WleHxvIqvmtkKkloyeM%3d**

291. Cahlan S, McCoy T, Samuels E, Traiano H. Visual timeline shows Bolsonaro flouted health recommendations before contracting coronavirus — and after. *Washington Post.* July 11, 2020. **https://www.washingtonpost.com/world/2020/07/11/bolsonaro-coronavirus-video-timeline/?arc404=true**

292. McCoy T, Traiano H. In the Brazilian Amazon, a sharp drop in coronavirus sparks questions over collective immunity. *Washington Post.* August 24, 2020. **https://www.washingtonpost.com/world/the_americas/brazil-coronavirus-manaus-herd-immunity/2020/08/23/0eccda40-d80e-11ea-930e-d88518c57dcc_story.html**

293. Hubler S, Fuller T, Singhvi A, Love J. Many Latinos couldn't stay home. Now virus cases are soaring in their communities. *New York Times.* June 26, 2020. **https://www.nytimes.com/2020/06/26/us/corona-virus-latinos.html**

294. Olivo A., Lang MJ, Harden JD. Crowded housing and essential jobs: why so many Latinos are getting coronavirus. *Washington Post.* May 26, 2020. **https://www.washingtonpost.com/local/latinos-coronavirus/2020/05/25/6b5c882a-946e-11ea-82b4-c8db161ff6e5_story.html**

295. Barrón-López L. 'So much worse than I ever thought it would be': Virus cases skyrocketing among Latinos. *Politico*. June 18, 2020. **https://www.politico.com/news/2020/06/18/rising-coronavirus-cases-among-latinos-alarm-public-health-experts-329248**

296. Sanchez-Guerra A, Jaramillo P, Latino E. "An alley without exit." Experts worry COVID-19 among Latinos will get dire without support. *News and Observer*. June 19, 2020. **https://www.newsobserver.com/news/coronavirus/article243618632.html** (And see **https://Covid-19.ncdhhs.gov/dashboard/cases**)

297. Stokes EK, Zambrano LD, Anderson KN, et al. Coronavirus Disease 2019 Case Surveillance — United States, January 22–May 30, 2020. *MMWR Morb Mortal Wkly Rep* 2020;69:759–765. DOI: **http://dx.doi.org/10.15585/mmwr.mm6924e2**

298. Chesin M. 'I've gone through so much pain already': Latino COVID-19 rates continue to rise. *Arizona Republic*. June 27, 2020. **https://www.azcentral.com/story/news/local/arizona-data/2020/06/27/latinocovid-19-rates-continue-rise/3263558001/**

299. Goldstein J. Did Floyd protests lead to a virus surge? Here's what we know. Epidemiologists have braced for a surge of coronavirus cases. But it has not come yet. *New York Times*. July 1, 2020. **https://www.nytimes.com/2020/07/01/nyregion/nyc-coronavirus-protests.html**

300. McCullough M. COVID-19 has not surged in cities with big protests, but it has in states that reopened early. Here are some possible reasons. *Inquirer*. June 27, 2020. **https://www.inquirer.com/health/coronavirus/coronavirus-no-spike-cities-despite-protests-big-surge-in-states-that-reopened-20200627.html**

301. Riga K. So…why hasn't there been a COVID spike from the protests? *TPM News*. June 24, 2020. **https://talkingpointsmemo.com/news/covid-spike-protest-testing-spread**

302. Balz D. Most Americans aren't buying Trump's rosy outlook on the coronavirus. *Washington Post*. July 9, 2020. **https://www.washingtonpost.com/news/powerpost/paloma/daily-202/2020/07/09/daily-202-most-americans-aren-t-buying-trump-s-rosy-outlook-on-the-coronavirus/5f0622fc88e0fa7b44f70856/?utm_campaign=wp_the_daily_202&utm_medium=email&utm_source=newsletter&wpisrc=nl_daily202**

303. Lederer E. UN says Latin America and Caribbean are COVID-19 `hot spot'. *Washington Post*. July 11, 2020. **https://www.washingtonpost.com/world/the_americas/un-says-latin-america-and-caribbean-are-covid-19-hot-spot/2020/07/09/77cf517c-c23c-11ea-8908-68a2b9eae9e0_story.html**

304. Harding A. Coronavirus in South Africa: Inside Port Elizabeth's 'hospitals of horrors'. *BBC News*. **https://www.bbc.com/news/world-africa-53396057**

305. Butler D. The ghost of influenza past and the hunt for a universal vaccine. Your first bout of flu may determine how you fare during the next pandemic. That's why scientists are trying to understand immunologic imprinting. *Nature*. August 8, 2018. **https://www.nature.com/articles/d41586-018-05889-1**

306. Lam TT, Shum MH, Zhu H, et al. Identifying SARS-CoV-2 related coronaviruses in Malayan pangolins. *Nature*. 2020. **https://doi.org/10.1038/s41586-020-2169-0 https://www.nature.com/articles/s41586-020-2169-0**

307. Quammen D. Did pangolin trafficking cause the coronavirus pandemic? *New Yorker*. August 24, 2020. **https://www.newyorker.com/magazine/2020/08/31/did-pangolins-start-the-coronavirus-pandemic**

Made in the USA
Middletown, DE
30 September 2020